TAKE IT OFF,
KEEP IT OFF

TAKE IT OFF, KEEP IT OFF

How I Went From Fat to Fit—
and You Can Too—
Safely, Effectively, and Permanently

FEATURING PJ'S PROVEN KO-90 PROGRAM

PAUL "PJ" JAMES

Da Capo
∞
LIFE
LONG

Da Capo Lifelong Books
A Member of the Perseus Books Group

Design and production by Brent Wilcox

Cataloging-in-Publication data for this book is available from the
Library of Congress.
First Da Capo Press edition 2012
ISBN 978-0-7382-1523-5 (paperback)
ISBN 978-0-7382-1574-7 (e-book)

Published by Da Capo Press
A Member of the Perseus Books Group
www.dacapopress.com

Note: The information in this book is true and complete to the best
of our knowledge. This book is intended only as an informative guide
for those wishing to know more about health issues. In no way is this
book intended to replace, countermand, or conflict with the advice
given to you by your own physician. The ultimate decision
concerning care should be made between you and your doctor. We
strongly recommend you follow his or her advice. Information in this
book is general and is offered with no guarantees on the part of the
authors or Da Capo Press. The authors and publisher disclaim all
liability in connection with the use of this book.

Da Capo Press books are available at special discounts for bulk
purchases in the U.S. by corporations, institutions, and other
organizations. For more information, please contact the Special
Markets Department at the Perseus Books Group, 2300 Chestnut
Street, Suite 200, Philadelphia, PA, 19103, or call (800) 810-4145,
ext. 5000, or e-mail special.markets@perseusbooks.com.

For every person who has made the commitment to get fit.
May you reach your goals and surpass all
expectations of what seems possible.

CONTENTS

INTRODUCTION

Give me ninety days, and I'll give you the rest of your life

When you find yourself eating your way through two large pizzas on the same day you vowed to kick off a dedicated six-month weight-loss plan, you know you're in serious trouble.

Unfortunately, that's precisely the sad situation I found myself in on July 1, 2009, after a pathetic five-minute workout that ended with my ankle giving out and my pride caving in. I was fat—264 pounds, to be exact. My cholesterol and blood-sugar levels were dangerously high, my lower back perpetually ached, and my inner thighs were forever chafed from rubbing against each other as I walked. Once an outgoing, adventurous go-getter, I'd begun holing up in bed, seeking solace in takeout burgers, fries, and pasta. My sex life with my girlfriend had imploded. I tried to put on a brave face when people teased me about my man boobs, but inside I was riddled with pain, frustration, and disgust. I knew I had to lose weight, but a terrible body image, rehab-worthy junk-food addiction, and nagging fear saddled me with doubt: What if I fail?

The kicker? Just six months earlier I had looked like this:

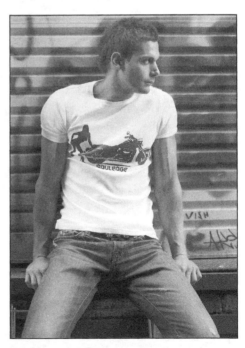

Believe it or not, that *is* me.

For nearly a decade I've worked as a sought-after personal trainer in Melbourne, Australia, and abroad helping hundreds of clients transform their bodies and, in the process, rediscover themselves. True, some of my regulars are aspiring bodybuilders and chiseled athletes, hell-bent on shredded abs and ripped quads. But for the most part my clientele is composed of people who are probably just like you: twenty to one hundred pounds overweight and desperately wanting to make a change. They don't need a butt you can bounce a quarter off of; they just want to be able to chase after their kids without panting for breath. Or fit in a pair of jeans from a mainstream store. Or bring their cholesterol levels down enough to get off medication.

Before I became a trainer I belonged to an even more body-conscious profession: high fashion/underwear modeling. I walked, bare chested, down catwalks for Dolce & Gabbana, Versace, Prada, Calvin Klein, and Jean Paul Gaultier. For a 264-pound man, that might sound horrifying, but when I was in my peak condition, it was the ultimate rush. Back then you truly could bounce a quarter off pretty much *any* part of my body! I lived for the spotlight, and the spotlight loved me back.

But when you're overweight or obese, you're forced to deal with an entirely different type of spotlight. People stare. Strangers judge. Labels like "lazy," "weak" and "disgusting" are hurtled in your direction, silently or out loud. The world assumes you simply lack willpower, that if you just buckled down and hit the gym, maybe turned down a cheeseburger here and there, you could shed the pounds.

You and I know better. We understand the power food wields—especially fatty, salty, or sugar-coated food. We've experienced the crippling body image issues that make joining a gym and working out in public seem impossible. We've been discriminated against for our looks, teased by family members and coworkers, mocked by the masses.

But if you've picked up this book, you're ready to change all that. You're ready to regain control of your addictive eating. You're ready to transform your body from an enemy into an ally. You're ready to seize hold of a life filled with excitement and joy and new adventures. You're ready to be healthy.

I will help you get there.

I have experienced life on both sides of the fence. In 2009 I embarked on a monumental journey in which I purposefully packed on 50 percent of my body weight in four months, then kept it on for another two. My inspiration: a growing number of overweight and obese personal-training clients who were coming to me seeking inspiration and empowerment. As someone who has always been intrigued by the human mind and who prides himself on an innate desire to help people, I felt helplessly ineffective. How could I truly relate to someone who couldn't walk for more than a block without getting winded or was terrified of stepping foot in a gym for fear of being stared at? I wanted—*needed*—to walk a mile in my heavy clients' shoes. And I arrogantly believed that both gaining and losing the weight would be a snap!

But the road from 6 percent to over 32 percent body fat was paved with confidence-sapping potholes and clinically depressed roadblocks. Being obese proved to be a terrifying existence for me. On one hand, I wanted to socialize with my friends and participate in hiking, swimming, and other outdoor activities that I've always loved. On the other hand, I was ashamed of my new physique and embarrassed about the person I had deteriorated into. The result was a vicious cycle that drove me to eat for comfort. I hid my emotions behind closed doors, with a pizza and a Coke to console me, and never wanted to leave.

Until I did.

The moment was slated to happen on July 1, 2009. As you now know, my mind and body had other plans. But despite my severely sprained ankle, newly acquired junk-food addiction, and wounded ego, there came a point when I felt compelled to break out of my overweight cage. When I realized that the joy and comfort that fatty, salty, sugary food provided was fleeting, dependably leaving me feeling disgusting and depressed. When I longed for the rush of a workout, the clean feeling of working up a good sweat, the pride of accomplishing a physical goal—even if it just meant walking on the treadmill for ten minutes. And that meant committing to change at all costs.

Getting back in shape was the single-most difficult challenge I have ever faced. The problem was that I feared I'd taken my weight gain too far and doubted my ability to change for the better. The desire to get in shape was barely there, and my cravings were so strong that I found controlling myself almost impossible. Add to that my self-imposed isolation: I refused to seek out extra assistance from those around me because I felt it was crucial that I faced every pain and emotion on my own so that, by the end of my lengthy experiment, I would have zero doubt that I could help anyone in the world.

But the fact is that I was far from alone on my journey. An astounding 68 percent of US adults—72 million Americans—are either overweight or obese.[1] Sixty percent of Americans are dieting at any given time and 220,000 Americans underwent bariatric surgery in 2009 alone.[2] Millions struggle with binge eating disorders and other dangerously unhealthy eating behaviors.[3] A recent survey found that young women have an average of thirteen brutal thoughts about their bodies every day—some as many as fifty or even one hundred—and 97 percent admitted to having at least one "I hate my body" moment (e.g., "You're bigger than her, fatty" and "Your stomach is fat; that is why you are alone").[4] Reality weight-loss TV shows like *The Biggest Loser, Dance Your Ass Off, Ruby, Celebrity Fit Club, DietTribe, Thintervention with Jackie Warner*, and *Honey, We're Killing the Kids* rule the airways. Fitness and diet books line bookstore shelves. Our world is sagging beneath an oversized population hell-bent on losing weight yet paralyzed by their own self-sabotaging behavior.

Today, a whopping 80 percent of my current clients start out overweight. But the difference between now and two years ago? I am in the unique position where I can discuss their lifestyle with intimate authority and firsthand knowledge. By picking up this book, you have hired me as *your* trainer too. Consider me your one-stop shop for getting into physical and emotional shape. I will outfit you with the top tools for building up your self-esteem, resetting your expectations, identifying and knocking down the weight-loss hurdles standing in your way, and respecting yourself enough to want to change. You'll learn how to move your body in new ways, building muscle and burning fat. I'll teach you how to prepare healthy, satisfying meals (I'm also a trained chef) to help you transition away from junk food and into simple, clean eating. And I'll encourage you to forgive yourself when you make mistakes, to allow yourself to feel happy, and to never give up. Your results will speak for themselves.

Whether you're intrigued by my journey and want an insider's take on life in an obese body, or if you're currently overweight, can't seem to figure out how to get into shape, and want to work with someone who's truly been there and knows your challenges firsthand, or even if you're in great shape but are seeking fresh moves and meals, welcome to *Take It Off, Keep It Off*. My motto: give me three months, and I'll give you back the rest of your life. I did it with my KO-90 program, and I'm going to help you do it too. If your desire is to lose weight and you've tried and tried again but with limited or no success, or even if this is your inaugural attempt, this book will provide the tools and skills you need to make that change. Put simply, if you have spent as long as you remember trying to lose weight and get in shape, it's time to acknowledge that what you're doing isn't working long term. It's time to start a new page and take your first real steps toward sustainable weight loss by replacing your old health habits once and for all. It's time to take control and accept responsibility for yourself.

I challenged myself to get inside obesity's head and untangle the drama and pitfalls associated with it. I undertook the journey so that I can offer a realistic approach to weight loss, one step at a time. Now, when I urge my clients to keep going, promising them that "Believe me, it does get easier," there's no comeback. Because I know . . . and it does. You have a choice. You just need to make it.

As your personal trainer, I'm going to introduce you to the exact plan that worked for me and a plan that continues to work for other people just like you. We'll tackle all the hard stuff—how your brain responds when you eat junk food, how to fuel your body optimally, how to do the most effective cardio and strength training moves, and finally how people just like you have succeeded in making their bodies their allies. But first, here's *my* story—and why I am so dedicated to helping you live the healthy, long, active life you deserve.

TAKE IT OFF,

PART I

FROM FIT TO FAT AND BACK

My Story of Gaining—and Losing—Half My Body Weight (and How That's Helped Me to Help You)

I entered the modeling world at the relatively ancient age of twenty-four. After spotting an untapped niche in underwear and fitness, I began experimenting with my diet and exercise routine. I may not have had the most chiseled cheekbones or the most masculine jaw, but I knew how to fuel and work my body to look a certain way. Some Australian modeling agencies rejected me, saying I didn't have the right "look." (Every time I'd ask them what that look was, and the only answer I got was, "It's hard to say, but it's not yours.") So in 2000 I took off for Japan, where I'd heard Western models like myself were more sought after. I celebrated my twenty-fourth birthday in Tokyo, which put me on par with industry veterans, not modeling newbies. But my outgoing personality and ability to be persistent without veering into obnoxiousness worked to my advantage, and what started off as a one-month working vacation bloomed into a six-year career.

I'm not going to lie: life was damn good as an underwear model. Gorgeous women were everywhere, I was invited to exclusive clubs, and I was paid a good amount of money basically to walk around in boxer briefs. But there were other models whose careers seemed to have taken off to another level. Physically speaking, they didn't appear to have anything more special, but they worked out harder and were financially rewarded for their commitment with more prestigious bookings.

While in Tokyo I was teaching English at a private school to earn some extra cash. Every day I'd take a dreadfully long, ninety-minute train ride each way to the school. My route took me past a large, white, windowless building—a gym—and one day, it just clicked: I needed to join. As an outdoors buff, I'd long avoided gyms because I didn't want to feel pinned down to treadmills and weight machines. But that day I realized that I could funnel my passion for exercise into *any* routine, especially when I knew there'd be a payoff at the end. The very next day I caught the train early so I could make a pit stop, and I signed myself up.

At first I felt completely lost in the gym, and the equipment intimidated me. But I began mimicking the routines of other guys whose physiques I admired, and soon enough I had their biceps and six-packs. My competitive edge emerged as I challenged myself to get stronger every day.

I also tapped into my background as a trained chef, cooking myself healthy meals like grilled fillet and steamed shitake mushrooms, or sea bass with ponzu sauce. I discovered a fantastic invention called a sushi train, a popular form of food presentation in Tokyo restaurants in which small plates of sushi and sashimi literally zoom around the table on a miniature train. The fish and rice offered the perfect protein-carb combination to fuel my workouts and, unlike my hometown of Melbourne, where a California Roll is more expensive than a DVD, these only cost 100 Yen, or about $1, per plate. Both my abs and my wallet were happy.

Eating "clean" (enjoying whole, unprocessed foods like fresh fruits and vegetables, whole grains and lean proteins instead of prepackaged items, fast food, or anything with a label) and working out—but never more than an hour a day—paid off, and my career continued to flourish. More exclusive jobs rolled in. But more importantly, my passion for fitness had been reignited, and I dreamt of returning home and making a name for myself in the Australian fitness industry. So in the beginning of 2006 I moved back to Melbourne to immerse myself in training with the goal of being able to work with *any* client and help my clients change their lives for the better.

At my gym back home strangers began approaching me—men as well as women—inquiring about my workout and eating regimens. Their interest humbled me, and I felt privileged to assume a sort of teaching role. Very quickly I discovered that I had a true passion for nutrition and fitness, and I realized that modeling itself wasn't what had given me such a rush; it was the hard, preparatory work and dedication put in at the gym and in the kitchen. I easily transitioned into my new job, helping others transform their bodies, and my newly found career began to take off.

BIG LOVE

I had found my passion, plain and simple, and it showed. Clients considered me approachable and easy to talk to, and I was honored to serve as their mentor and motivator. As word spread, my clientele expanded—both literally and figuratively—as more and more overweight and obese men and women sought me out. No longer was I only helping regular gymgoers; these were people who had serious weight to lose—along with all the baggage that comes with that territory. An emotional and physical disconnect quickly manifested itself: whereas I could train my fit or semifit clients with my eyes shut, I had no idea how to respond when a heavy client claimed he simply couldn't muster the energy to walk for five minutes on the treadmill or tried to explain how anxious and embarrassed she felt in a gym environment. As someone who subsisted on egg whites, grilled fish, steamed sweet potatoes, and broccoli, I hadn't the slightest clue about life as an emotional eater, junk-food addict, or gymophobe. I found myself doling out general advice—"Do more cardio" or "Eat less fatty foods"—and they responded with, "You're a freaking underwear model! You have no clue what it's like for us." What could I say? They were right: I *didn't* know.

Now—not to sound corny—empathy is one of the core principles by which I live my life. I know people don't typically correlate the words "underwear model" and "compassion," but ever since my seventh-grade English teacher, Mrs. John, taught us the definition of empathy, I've felt an affinity toward the concept—so much so that I had the word tattooed inside my left wrist at age twenty-eight.

But for the first time in years I felt like I couldn't empathize. I didn't have an answer for my clients. Their questions tossed me far outside my comfort zone and I felt almost reluctant to train them, like I was doing them a disservice. On a very basic and essential level, I couldn't understand how difficult it was for an overweight person to get into shape, and had no clue as to the best approach to help them mend their eating habits.

THE ANTI—NEW YEAR'S RESOLUTION

Around that time, I had read—and been blown away by—a study that said 67 percent of Australian adults were overweight or obese. As a nation, we were fast approaching the United States, where the numbers were just as depressing: a mind-boggling 68 percent of US adults fall into those weight categories.[1] It would have been far easier to ignore the numbers and simply build a roster full of fit or semi-fit clients, but I felt that I ought to be able to help anyone who approached me, regardless of their weight. And the idea for *Take It Off, Keep It Off* was born.

In order to empathize truly with my clients, I had to do something drastic—something that would allow me literally to walk in their shoes and experience life as an overweight individual. Half-hearted weight gain and a part-time gym membership wouldn't cut it; I knew total immersion was the only way to understand. If I wanted to return to my clients with authentic knowledge of obesity's physical frustrations and emotional aches and pains, I'd have to take myself to my limits. With that realization, I decided that I would aim to pack on half my body weight in three months, maintain it for three additional months, and then take it off before the year was through. Imagine *The Biggest Loser* but in reverse.

I was confident that I'd be able to walk away having gained a real sense of empathy and would be able to prove that, with dedication and the proper tools, weight loss success *is* possible. Not once did I anticipate that my little experiment would have life-altering physical and emotional repercussions, from fat accumulation around my internal organs to a bout with depression to a deep-dish addiction that nearly did me in.

GET BIG OR GO HOME

I kicked off my journey on New Year's Eve, December 31, 2008, intent on adding nearly 100 pounds of flab to my 176-pound, 6 percent body-fat frame. Most people ring in the New Year by planting a passionate kiss on their partner; I breezed past my now-fiancée, Lisa, to undertake a full-scale binge. My first fat-bomb meal included four lamb gyros, a heaping plate of BBQ, salad, bread and dips, plus a platter of fried fish for dessert . . . all washed down by eight cans of Coca-Cola. My body, used to asparagus and egg whites, was so confused by the sudden influx of grease and salt that I gained ten pounds overnight (primarily water weight).

For two weeks I was in hog heaven. The tuna sashimi and steamed rice that kept me fueled and fat-free in Tokyo were swiftly replaced with cheeseburgers and powdered donuts with Fanta chasers. Foods normally reserved for my Saturday "cheat day" were now up for grabs 24–7: bubbly mac and cheese, crispy buckets of KFC's finest, savory ramen noodles, caramel ice cream, and fudge-drizzled dessert pizzas. My buddy David owns a pizza joint called Crisp, and he'd host me for weekly all-you-can-eat dinner sessions. In the mornings I toasted the rising sun with three liters of chocolate milk, scrambled eggs, and jam-slathered bread. At night, I would polish off an entire roast chicken before hitting the sack. Then I'd wake up and do it all again. Meanwhile, I reduced my energy expenditure to nearly zero—no lifting weights, no swimming in the ocean, no Sunday golf outings. I dedicated myself to being a professional couch potato.

It wasn't long before word of my "Hunk to Chunk" metamorphosis caught on. Members of my gym set up a donation box, in which they would deposit hi-cal offerings for me to gorge on. One member told my friend, a reporter from a local paper, about the endeavor, and within days, I had landed on the front of *The Herald Sun*, one of Australia's most popular newspapers. Camera crews camped outside the gym, and three major TV networks vied for an interview. The United States, where gastric bypass surgery and anticellulite treatments reign supreme, took notice too; *ESPN, ABC News, Good Morning America, Inside Edition, Fox and Friends, The Doctors*, and *E! News* all came knocking. Photos of my stomach, which by Month Three rivaled a full-term pregnant woman's belly, went viral.

DOES MY LIVER LOOK FAT IN THIS?

But it wasn't all bacon double cheeseburgers and deep-fried mozzarella sticks. Having a "Get Out of Diet-Jail Free" card might sound exhilarating, but the novelty quickly wore off, as I saw my years of hard work—my very livelihood—start to disintegrate. The daily routine—gorging on breakfast, training clients, returning home for an early lunch, taking a nap, consuming lunch number two, watching TV, and preparing for a gigantic dinner—was taking its toll. I had traded lat pull-downs for ham-and-cheese roll-ups, and as a result, I watched as my deltoids vanished beneath a duvet of fat. Normally buzzing with energy, I grew lethargic, unmotivated, and dejected. I stopped socializing. My sex life all but vanished. Motivating clients to get in shape while I was falling out of it proved to be a complicated psychological struggle.

If you're wondering how clients reacted to my little endeavor, the answer—somewhat surprisingly—is: extremely well. They thought it was fantastic that someone would go to such lengths to walk a mile in their shoes, and I found that the heavier I became, the harder they worked and the cleaner they ate. It's almost as if seeing me balloon before their eyes was the perfect motivation for them *not* to look like that. The reaction from prospective clients wasn't quite the same. Imagine walking into a gym and enquiring about personal training, only to be pointed in the direction of a guy who looked like he was training to be a sumo wrestler!

Before diving into my first bucket of fried chicken, however, I'd consulted with a physician, Steve Daniel, MD. I wanted to know if the negative health effects I was sure to incur—elevated cholesterol and blood sugar, increased heart rate—would be reversible. He explained that the more my waistline expanded, the more I'd be opening myself up to the risk of a heart attack, Type 2 diabetes, and metabolic syndrome. But although he couldn't guarantee my safety, Dr. Daniel felt that, with my fitness history and commitment to losing the weight within the year, I needn't worry too much about long-term damage from my get-big-or-go-home plan.

Sure enough, within the first few months of the experiment my cholesterol and blood sugar skyrocketed, and fat began to take up residence around my liver. Stretch marks tore through my skin as it strained to contain my new moobs (man boobs) and muffin top. Friends teased me mercilessly for walking like a duck (in an effort to spare my chafing inner-thigh skin). As my gut ballooned, a visible arch developed in my spine as it bowed under the excess weight. A dearth of fresh produce left me plagued with colds. My ankles were perpetually swollen, and my sleep sucked.

By the fourth month Dr. Daniel was strongly encouraging me to stop, both for my physical health and my emotional well-being. My depression symptoms raised red flags, and my cholesterol, blood sugar, and liver enzymes were showing no signs of backing down. My physical therapist was worried that my spine would not straighten back out. Lisa was begging me to quit—nobody wants to see their loved ones suffer, especially when that suffering is elective. But by that point there had already been a good amount of publicity surrounding my experiment, so I felt like I'd be letting everyone down. I wanted to experience those thoughts and feelings, no matter how disturbing they might be. Stopping two months short was not an option.

"FROM GREEK ADONIS TO HOMER SIMPSON"

I arrived at my goal weight of 264 pounds feeling miserably dejected and struggling to identify with the person I had become. The man who once earned a living baring his body in front of the camera now found himself hiding beneath blankets in bed, seeking solace in takeout and reality TV. Like the six million other Americans who binge eat,[2] I had begun turning to food for comfort. The fact is that although I had anticipated the health risks and medical repercussions of this experiment, I had vastly underestimated—if not entirely dismissed—its potential impact on my psyche.

Meanwhile, the world—not to mention the very clients who inspired my project—was watching. Critics early on, who deemed my "Fit to Fat and Back" experiment nothing more than a publicity stunt, stood by, waiting to pounce on any perceived failure. And though I initially had welcomed the media attention for its ability to raise the public's consciousness surrounding obesity, maintaining a positive self-image is difficult when headlines about you are screaming, "From Greek Adonis to Homer Simpson!" and "Nightmare on Fat Street," regardless of whether you gained weight purposefully or not. My friends teased me about my newly formed man boobs, from which a once-fierce nipple piercing now dangled pathetically. I wore a size-46 belt.

The road back to fitness would prove even more challenging, as I quickly realized that losing weight would be much harder to deal with than I'd ever envisioned. Depression, back pain, loose skin, stretch marks, self-doubt, and embarrassment were just some of the issues with which I wrestled. Despite my years of dedicated workouts, I doubted my ability to shed the pounds. I was fighting strong cravings and addictions, feelings of hopelessness, and a real loss of identity. My confidence was sapped.

Rock bottom hit on June 30, 2009, the day before my first official day back at the gym. *The Herald Sun* wanted to attend my first training session. We met at a local park, where I took my shirt off (the media was really milking the whole "man boob" thing) and stretched a few lingering muscles. The cameraman asked me if I could jog into frame as they filmed some shots. I put on a smile, made it about ten feet, and twisted my right ankle. The joints and ligaments simply couldn't handle the excess weight, and my ankle ballooned up immediately, foreshadowing a three-month injury.

Embarrassed, ashamed, and feeling sorry for myself, I returned to the gym. I told the documentary team that had been following me that I wanted to be left alone; after they had left, I picked up the phone and ordered two large pizzas. This was emotional eating at its purest, most elemental form. The pies arrived, and as I dug in, I heard noise coming from outside the gym kitchen. Little did I know my camera crew had returned for a piece of equipment they'd left behind. I was busted, pepperoni in hand.

WHAT GOES UP MUST COME DOWN

What a frigging wreck I was! I felt defeated, like I'd let all my clients down. Six months earlier my body functioned as a well-oiled machine, burning through clean food and showing results after every weight-lifting session. But when you're obese, you can spend an entire day in the gym and not notice any changes. All you notice is that you're hungry. (And I *was*, in fact, obese: my body fat had now topped out beyond 32 percent, which, according to the American Council on Exercise, is a full 7 percent *above* the minimum guidelines for obesity.)[3] I was too ashamed to do the final Dexa scan to measure my exact body fat percentage at 264 pounds, but it was probably over 35 percent.

When I was fit, I had just assumed that, come July 1, I'd be itching to get back in the gym and resume working out. I couldn't have been further from the truth. I was embarrassed to go out in public, let alone in workout gear. My food cravings had shifted so swiftly that it was mind-numbing. I had leapt from leafy greens to Dairy Queen, and my taste buds didn't want to take the long trip back.

That's not shocking, considering the true addictive potential of junk food. Research shows that when humans consume fattening foods, our brains react as they would if we were snorting cocaine. Pleasure receptors in the brain light up, "hooking" us on

Snickers and fried chicken.[4] When I indulged in malted milkshakes and cheese fries, my mind acted much like that of a drug addict, and I felt powerless to fight it.

People always ask me how I picked myself up and got over that six-month hump. What it came down to was this: I didn't accept the person I had become, physically or emotionally, and I was determined to change that. I now hated the way working out made me feel, but I hated the way I felt *not* working out even more. "This is just a stepping stone to feeling good," I kept repeating. Whether I would reach my goal in six months was anyone's guess, but I promised myself, over and over, that it *would* happen.

Whittling my keg back down to a six-pack seemed like a mission impossible, so I started with baby steps. I assured myself, "You just have to make it to the gym every day." That's it. Not: "You must log three miles on the Elliptical today" or "You need to lift weights for forty-five minutes." Simply showing up was good enough, and that turned out to be half the battle. Sure, I was sore, exhausted, and unable to eke out even the most basic of moves like push-ups or crunches, but knowing that all I needed to do was show up kept me going. *That* I could do. Once I arrived at the gym, I realized I might as well work out or else I was just wasting time and energy. Watching others train triggered an urge inside, reminding me how good being in shape used to feel.

What began as baby steps would eventually evolve into giant strides. Within my first week back I was sleeping better and my lower back wasn't aching as badly. The results weren't groundbreaking, but I was taking a step in the right direction.

The addictions were a bit trickier to kick. I had grown accustomed to soothing myself with food. Chicken nuggets and mashed potatoes filled me up and comforted me. Ice cream numbed the pain of feeling disgusting. But I had to look deep inside myself and face the fact that all of that junk only made me feel better for about ten minutes; after that the sadness and disgust crept back in—only now they were compounded by an overstuffed stomach. All of that so-called delicious food left me with a horrible taste in my mouth, literally and figuratively, and I decided I needed to change.

The truth was that when I ate well for a few days, I was instantly rewarded with positive results in my mood, shape, and skin clarity. When I abused my body with bad food for a few days, I fell into a slump, dreading crawling out of bed in the morning and hating the world.

After weighing up all these emotions, I knew that even though overcoming my food addictions was challenging at the best of times, I needed to turn my life around. That meant removing temptations by cleaning out my cupboards, trashing every sleeve of cookies and six-pack of beer. I went to sleep at an hour that allowed me to wake up feeling energized. At every meal I drank two glasses of water. I created a vision board

(What? You thought Oprah cornered that market?) with inspirational sayings and photos and hung it where I would see it every morning and evening—that made the goal seem vital and realistic.

Taking responsibility for myself had a snowball effect: when I stopped eating crap, I felt healthier. When I felt healthier, I had more energy to exercise. The more I worked out, the faster I saw results, and this reinforced my commitment to clean eating. And it all started with two conscious decisions: one was to stop ordering fries with everything and the other was to shave off the unkempt beard I had been sporting for the last five months.

I knew I was going to have slip-ups along the way, and I promised myself I'd treat myself kindly when I did. (That promise, however, proved quite difficult to keep; I often bashed myself for slipping up, punishing myself with more reckless eating.) Even so, I knew that even if I could only handle making one dietary tweak a day, those improvements would add up, and eventually, I'd overcome this beast.

By Month Ten (four months back into my routine) I was seeing noticeable results. My relationship with friends and with Lisa had improved—mostly because I wasn't a miserable mope all the time. Shades of my old outgoing personality reemerged, and I found myself joking more and making new plans. My client relationships grew stronger. Even modest changes, like shaving an inch off my waist, would instill a boatload of confidence. And the more confidence I gained, the more driven I became to keep going. All of the good stuff snowballed, and by December 23, 2009, I was back down to my original weight of 176 pounds. Two months later I shot the cover of *Men's Fitness*.

GETTING BACK ON TRACK

This book—and the journey that inspired it—was born out of a genuine desire to see how "the other half" lives. I've walked a mile in an obese person's shoes, and I kept walking until those last few stubborn pounds came off. My success is proof that *it is possible* for everyone to lose weight in a healthy manner. You might not aspire to walk down a runway in your underwear, glistening in oil, but what about walking down the street, brimming with confidence? I don't claim that I have experienced exactly what it feels like to be overweight all your life, but I have definitely gained a real insight into the psychological, emotional, and physical effects obesity has on the individual—and for that I am truly thankful.

Today, my clients know *I know* what it feels like to be terrified of failing. To be embarrassed to exercise in public. To be intimidated by the gym. To be ashamed of the way I look. I've successfully bridged the gap between fit and fat, and as a result, clients are more receptive. Their newfound openness shines in their results. They respect the sacrifices I made and feel comfortable enough to trust me with their lives. *That* is the ultimate reward.

Use *Take It Off, Keep It Off* as an opportunity to change. Of course, everyone's weight-loss goal is different—you may want to lose ten pounds, you may want to lose one hundred. My goal is to help you do it in a manner that's safe, effective—and permanent. Make a commitment to get healthy and push yourself to follow through. Healthy weight loss is like a freight train: once you start feeling good about yourself, there's no stopping.

PART 2

GETTING STARTED

The KO-90 Game Plan

In your hands you hold the key to unlocking your weight-loss goals. This is the same plan I myself followed as I shed 50 percent of my body weight, and I still rely on it to this day to stay fit, healthy, and buzzing with energy. Here are my secrets; as you'll see, there are no tricks or gimmicks—just a plan that's straightforward, safe, and effective:

A. Every day, before I even think about breakfast, I kick things off with fifteen minutes of cardio.

B. I fuel myself with three meals, two snacks, and plenty of water.

C. Four days a week I dedicate fifty minutes to lifting weights.

That's it. No soul-sucking, hour-long Stairmaster sessions. No starvation. No need to set up a cot at the gym. This is how I originally maintained my 6 percent body fat status, and it got me back there after I'd ballooned beyond 32 percent.

GIVE ME THREE MONTHS AND I'LL GIVE YOU BACK THE REST OF YOUR LIFE

The KO-90 plan is a three-month system designed to reshape both your body and mind. I worked hard to knock out those ninety pounds I'd put on; I decided to call the program that helped me shed the weight (and keep it off) the KO-90 plan. Your weight loss will vary according to your own personal needs and goals—but this plan will work whether you want to lose nine or ninety pounds. Your key focus will be fat loss as opposed to just weight loss. Focus on body shape rather than body weight, and you will transform your body beyond what you thought was possible. Within three months you should be able to lose about 12 to 24 percent of your body weight (that's 1 to 2 percent per week—the greater your starting weight, the more pounds you can safely lose per week without sacrificing muscle). At that point, if you still have more weight to lose, you'll simply continue the clean eating and exercise regimen outlined in these pages. If you've already reached your goal by the three-month milestone, you can transition to the Maintenance Plan (page 95). Like anything worthwhile in life—our friendships, love lives, children, jobs—it will require hard work and dedication. The first month will be challenging. But the payoff will be the chance to live the life you want—and deserve. Three months to revolutionize your life? That's a worthwhile investment.

Throughout the book you'll be hearing from some of the amazing people I've worked with—people just like you who've wanted to change and have done it. If you're looking for additional inspiration or want to hear more from people who've worked with me—what really worked for them and how it can work for you too—skip to the final chapter and read more.

The KO-90 plan is based on six fundamental concepts. Allow me to introduce you to . . .

THE GAME CHANGERS

#1: Fat Loss Trumps Weight Loss

"But aren't they the same thing?" you might be asking. Not in the slightest. When weight loss is your main priority, all you care about is seeing the number on the scale plummet. The most popular reality TV shows, which follow obese individuals as they work out for eight hours a day to the point of exhaustion, focus on weight loss: getting that number to drop from 298 one week to 280 the next. But just because the digits are taking a nosedive, it doesn't mean you're losing fat—and fat is what gets you into trouble with heart disease, stroke, diabetes, cancer, and more.

PJ's Pointer

Gimme 1 Percent

Rather than focusing on pounds lost per week, aim to shed 1 percent of your total body weight per week.

Popular diets and the media glorify individuals who shed the most amount of weight in the shortest amount of time, typically by combining massive amounts of cardio with harsh calorie restriction. And yes, you will lose a seemingly glorious amount of weight (much of it water)—at first. But you're setting yourself up for

When a client decides to lose weight, I ask them, "Is this your number-one priority in life?" If weight loss is way down on your list—or even if it's number three or number four—you're not ready. There needs to be an urgency to make the change—and make it *now*. That motivation might be an upsetting, weight-related medical diagnosis, a particularly jarring comment from a friend or stranger (e.g., "When are you expecting?" . . . when you're not), a doctor's urging, or an embarrassing situation (e.g., you started having chest pains while attempting to play tag with your kids). The pain has to be so strong that you simply cannot live in your condition any longer—you're at rock bottom. When that's the case, you'll be truly open to making a change.

failure by adopting a severe plan that will likely be impossible to stick to and will just leave you frustrated and feeling like a failure. Unless you're an Olympian whose job is to dedicate your entire work day to training, your life simply isn't set up to support such extreme exercise. And if you *were* an Olympic athlete, you'd be eating adequate calories to power you through your marathon workouts.

By focusing on fat loss, you'll be setting yourself up for a lifetime of success. If you adhere to Game Changer #1, you will not step on the scale and find you've lost a mind-blowing amount of weight at the end of every week (though you very well may lose up to 10 pounds in the first week, mostly water loss). More realistically, you'll shed between 1 to 2 percent of your body weight every week. So if you weigh 250 pounds, you'll lose between 2.5 to 5 pounds per week; if you weigh 175 pounds, you'll lose between 1.75 to 3.5 pounds per week. That doesn't look as sexy as the huge numbers they pull off on reality TV shows, but it's a steady, maintainable amount—one that's realistic and will help with long-term health.

A fat loss focus will also manifest itself with significant changes in your body shape. Weight lifting will build your muscles, which will begin to show their face as you slowly melt away the layer of fat blanketing them. I will never forget flexing my biceps three months into my workout routine and seeing that they actually pointed upward instead of seeing my triceps just sagging downward. Now *that* was a motivating day.

#2: Success = 70 Percent Nutrition, 30 Percent Fitness

The majority of your weight loss is going to take place *outside* the gym. Don't get me wrong: weights and cardio are crucial to your success. But you can spend hours on the

Elliptical machine or Spin bike and remain overweight if you fail to gain control of your eating.

In our society we associate hard work with rewards. If you spend eternity (or what seems like it) on the treadmill, you're surely protected from a harmless little hamburger, right? Absolutely not. When it comes to burning fat, the story changes a bit. Yes, you still need to work hard, but in different areas. Fat loss is a simple equation: burn off more fat than you consume. Eating clean—minimizing sodium, fat, and carbs and sticking with whole, natural foods like leafy greens, lean meats, and whole grains—allows the body to burn stored fat. You cannot succumb to the "Oh, it's just this once" mentality—"Oh, it's just one ice cream cone" or "Oh, it's only one donut." That donut never exists in a vacuum—it's bound to turn into "just one" beer at a concert plus "just one" slice of pizza at book club. You can easily wipe out forty-five minutes of a sweat-soaked gym session with half of a toasted bagel and cream cheese. Any and all of these will rob you of a real shot at achieving a healthy weight. So realize the critical importance of eating clean.

Then, devote yourself to fifteen minutes of interval-based cardio per day, done at specific times and under specific conditions, to blast fat. (More on this later.) With the KO-90 plan cardio is always done first thing in the morning, before you've eaten, to maximize your system's fat-burning potential. I know, I know: you're too tired to wake up early and workout. You're hungry when you first wake up and will faint if you don't eat something before exercising. I used these same excuses too when I was trying to get back in shape. And the truth is that I *was* tired. I *was* hungry. But those feelings weren't limited to the early morning hours. Overweight and obese people are forever tired and hungry because we're sabotaging ourselves with our actions. Think of your thin friends: are they constantly exhausted and always talking or thinking about their next meal? Not likely. They're probably full of energy and always running around from work to the gym to their family and friends, enjoying an active lifestyle and eating in moderation. Well, they didn't just luck into that lifestyle (not most of them, anyway). You pave your own path. Like begets like: eat healthy, feel healthy. Workout and avoid weight gain. And although fifteen minutes may seem like a lot at first, you'll be surprised at how it becomes totally doable—and you may actually enjoy it!

Strength training is the third crucial component that will set you on the path to becoming lean. Lifting weights promotes toning and definition, and after adding this to your cardio and healthy eating, you will be unstoppable . . . and so will the fat loss!

Would you rather eat smart and devote fifteen minutes a day to cardio, knowing you're treating your body well and setting yourself up for success? Or would you rather eat whatever and whenever you like and (fruitlessly) attempt to burn the food off by

Resist the urge to snack on poor food choices. You will not die if you don't try the cupcakes your coworker baked. You will not spiral into a depression if you pass on the fries everyone else is scarfing down. You need to reframe your mindset: instead of thinking, "I'll never be able to eat a cheeseburger again!," ask yourself, "Do I *really* need this right now? Will it kill me to skip it?"—and remind yourself that this is not the last burger/cupcake/plate of fries on earth. There will always be more.

dragging yourself through endless hours of cardio? I know what I prefer. The first example taps into stored fat and begins to change your body inside and out. The second example is a form of defeated acceptance and self-serving justification of poor eating habits. All it does is cause you to become frustrated, obsessed with food, and disappointed with your lack of progress in weight, shape, and mood.

If you eat well from day one and train specifically for fat loss by following the KO-90 plan, you will see results in the first week. Day after day, week after week, it will become easier, until one morning, waking up at 6 a.m. to hit the pavement will feel like second nature, as will be returning home for a breakfast of hearty oatmeal and a steaming mug of black coffee or tea. You won't even think about what you're doing anymore: it will just be another day . . . but what a healthy day it will be! Get your clean eating down pat, and the weight will start to come off. Stay on track. It's okay to feel your stomach gurgling—think of it as the sound of your metabolism igniting! Resist the urge to snack on poor food choices. You do not need or deserve immediate gratification. Burning fat off that you just consumed will leave you in exactly the same place, day after day—overweight and undermotivated. I'm guessing this hasn't worked for you in the past. If you're reading this book, that tells me you're no longer interested in maintaining the status quo and you no longer

SUCCESS STORY DORA

"I had tried other trainers, but it was like we were speaking different languages. One trainer wanted to start by going for a run at the park; he didn't understand how daunting and difficult that seemed for me at 374 pounds. PJ understood how hard it really was and that when you are heavy, you have joint pain, swollen feet, and can't run."

—Dora Dogas, age thirty-five, lost 198 pounds . . . and counting

accept the person you see in the mirror. Break the cycle and replace bad habits with smart habits. Soon your friends and family will notice a difference in how you look and act, but, more importantly, so will you. Change is incredibly inspirational and unbelievably motivating. My clients get encouraged by positive changes like dropping a pant

SUCCESS STORY Z O I

"PJ changed my life by giving me the know-how I need for a healthy lifestyle. He could leave for a year and I'd still do my gym routine and make the right food choices. I'll live by these guidelines for the rest of my life: once you learn to ride a bike, you don't forget it!"

—Zoi Georgiou, age twenty-five, lost 55 pounds

SUCCESS STORY B e r n a d e t t e

"PJ taught me that anyone can be a size ten."

—Bernadette Clarebrough, age fifty-one, lost 53 pounds

size or feeling strong enough to resist the bread basket at a restaurant, and those changes spur them on to continue to eat and train well. Once a person sees results, it's very hard to give in and quit. It really is up to you.

Still having a hard time saying no to your favorite indulgences? This should turn you off: Check out how long it takes to burn off a single donut or burger*:

To burn off: McDonald's BigMac®, large fries, hot fudge sundae, large Coke: 1,680 calories

It takes: 2 hours, 27 minutes of running (at 5 mph)

To burn off: Dunkin' Donuts Blueberry Crumb Donut and large Vanilla Bean Coolata®: 1,360 calories

It takes: 4 hours, 48 minutes of walking (at 3 mph)

To burn off: Wendy's Baconator® Double and large Chocolate Fudge Frosty Shake: 1,480 calories

It takes: 2 hours, 28 minutes of swimming freestyle (slow/moderate pace)

To burn off: Pizza Hut Hand-Tossed Style MeatLovers Pizza® (three slices): 900 calories

It takes: 1 hour, 45 minutes of biking (at 10–12 mph)

To burn off: Large Dairy Queen Cookie Dough Blizzard®: 1,300 calories

It takes: 2 hours, 10 minutes of tennis

To burn off: Taco Bell Volcano Nachos® with ground beef, beans, nacho cheese, cheesy molten hot lava sauce, and reduced-fat sour cream: 980 calories

It takes: 4 hours, 35 minutes of Hatha yoga

To burn off: Starbucks Java Chip Frappuccino® and raspberry scone: 940 calories

It takes: Just over 1 hour on the Elliptical (medium pace)

To burn off: IHOP Simple & Fit Three Eggs and Pancakes® w/hash browns with four pork sausage links: 1,480 calories

It takes: 19 hours, 13 minutes of sleeping (!)

*All estimates are for a person weighing 180 pounds.

#3: Follow the 60/30/10 Plan

Those numbers refer to the KO-90 plan ratio of protein to carbohydrates to fat, and I'm willing to bet a massive sum of money that it's wildly different from your current plan. I know, because it's one that, despite following it myself throughout my twenties, I absolutely balked at when forced to confront it in an effort to lose weight. But by reducing the amount of dietary carbohydrates, you'll be teaching your body to tap into stored fat for energy. And because you'll be consuming a larger amount of protein, you'll fuel and maintain muscle mass.

Lean protein will rule, along with healthy doses of energy-sustaining carbs and a small amount of essential fats. You'll be asked to remove all dairy, fruit, added sugar, added salt and alcohol for the first twelve weeks. I know that probably translates in your head as "Eliminate all fun, pleasure, and taste from your life," but the fact is that we have become so accustomed—if not addicted—to salty, greasy, sugary junk food that we barely even recognize real food anymore. Even a seemingly virtuous food can harbor an embarrassing amount of garbage. For instance, McDonald's oatmeal manages to pack more sugar than a Snickers bar and only ten fewer calories than an Egg McMuffin or cheeseburger.[1]

In this plan lean, muscle-fueling protein will become your new best friend. Think fillet or flank steak, grilled skinless chicken breast, tilapia, cod, flounder, and tofu. Oils and other fats will make guest appearances but only in the form of heart-healthy fats, like a few avocado chunks sprinkled into a salad or a drizzle of flaxseed oil on your roasted asparagus. I'll encourage you to drink a decent amount of water and herbal tea in order to curb hunger and keep your body hydrated.

Please trust me and allow yourself to commit to this plan, even though it might be a little more regimented than what you're used to. It's only twelve weeks. That's *nothing* compared to the promise of a longer, healthier life. After the first three months have passed you'll have the option to loosen things up a bit and transition to a 50/40/10 protocol, with the occasional "bad meat" being allowed. But you might find that the 60/30/10 ratio works so well for you that you want to stick with it. After all, you will actually be eating like the way we were meant to eat. I know it sounds doubtful now, but wait and see—you might surprise yourself.

Here are some other key facets of the nutritional plan (these will be covered in greater detail in Part 4):

Keep it clean. This means tossing out pretty much anything with a label or wrapper and choosing whole, natural foods, like vegetables, lean meats, and grains. You'll accomplish this by shopping the perimeter of your grocery store, frequenting farmer's markets and avoiding anything with more than a few ingredients or an ingredient you cannot pronounce (Sodium tripolyphosphate or powdered cellulose, anyone?).

Always eat breakfast. Do this after your morning workout, not before.

Pile on the produce. You'll get to experiment with all manner of vegetables, making sure they take up at least half of your plate at lunch and dinner. Leafy green veggies, like spinach and kale, are especially nutrient dense while also delivering minimal calories.

Fuel up with sustainable carbs. You won't need sugary soda or candy to make it through the 3 p.m. slump when your body's humming along on natural fuel, like oatmeal, baked sweet potatoes, or whole-grain couscous.

PJ's
Pointer

I know what you're thinking: how can I give up alcohol when just *reading* about all of this hard work makes me want to drink? But my clients—even the most die-hard oenophiles—are amazed at how nearly every area of their life improves when they quit drinking, even for only a few months. Nearly instantly, they start sleeping more soundly. They shed fat more easily because they're not swallowing hundreds of chemically laden, liquid calories. And they make smarter eating choices when booze isn't weakening their willpower. While modeling in Europe and Asia I made it through a three-year period when I didn't take a single drink. If I can endure Gucci and Prada parties with no champagne, you can turn down a Happy Hour martini.

"My whole attitude about eating and drinking has changed dramatically. Quantity has given way to quality. I no longer desire to eat the mountains of food that I used to. And I don't even think about red wine anymore. If you had told me three months ago that I would enjoy black tea or coffee without sugar or milk, I would have said, 'That's BS.' But now, I enjoy eating clean food—I actually look forward to it."

—Andrew Fedorowicz, age sixty-two, lost 48 pounds . . . and counting

#4: Lift Weight to Drop Weight

Bottom line: strength training is where it's at. I'm sure the cardio room at your gym overflows with people slogging away on treadmills, Stairmasters, and bikes—and don't get me wrong: cardio has its place. (See Game Changer #5). But pumping iron torches fat and calories and will push you toward your goal more efficiently than spending hours circling the track.

Here's why it works: fat hardly burns at all when you rest. It just sits there, clogging your arteries and keeping you in plus-sized pants. Muscle, however, is metabolically active all the time, even when you're sleeping. Your body uses about 4.5 to 7 calories per pound of muscle every day. That means if a 220-pound man with 30 percent body fat increases his muscle mass and lowers his body fat to 25 percent, he'll burn an additional 50 to 83 calories per day at rest simply by adding muscle. If a 180-pound woman with 30 percent body fat increases her muscle mass and lowers her body fat to 25 percent, she'll burn an additional 41 to 63 calories per day at rest. The number on their scales might not go down, but their body composition will change entirely . . . for the better.

Some other reasons lifting weights rocks:

- You'll have more endurance.
- You'll prevent injuries.
- You'll strengthen your bones.
- You'll reduce your risk of developing Type 2 diabetes.
- You'll sleep better.
- You'll fight age and gravity.

#5: Keep Cardio Under Control

I see a lot of overweight gym members sweating it out on the treadmill for sixty to ninety minutes a day, sometimes longer. They're playing into the widely held belief that you have to sweat buckets to burn fat, that the harder and faster you go, the more fat you will burn. But contrary to our cardio-crazed culture's beliefs, you need not spend hour after hour running, biking, Ellipticizing, or aerobicizing. I know it seems to defy logic, but fat loss actually occurs at a *lower* heart rate, and it can be done in just fifteen minutes per day.

Heart-pumping cardiovascular exercise will complement your strength training and ramp up fat loss. You'll also experience those sought-after endorphin rushes and be able to clean up little dietary mistakes you make along the way, like picking fries off a friend's plate. My clients experience optimal results with only thirty minutes of cardio per day (fifteen in the morning and a fifteen-minute walk after dinner) plus two to four fifty-minute weight lifting sessions per week.

My rule with cardio is simple and it applies to all overweight people: fifteen minutes of interval training (either on the Elliptical or by walking outside), alternating one minute at a fast pace and one minute at about 60 percent capacity. Cardio should always be done on an empty stomach and first thing in the morning—that is, it should be the first thing on your mind when you wake up. This is called "fasted training," and it's been shown to prevent weight gain.[2]

You don't have to rush to the gym: throw on a T-shirt and shorts and head outdoors for a walk around your neighborhood. (The more overweight you are, in order to prevent injuries, the less I encourage running.) You'll be done in the time it takes to hit the snooze button three times, and you can shower and head to work fueled by a sense of accomplishment and a jolt of natural energy.

#6: I Did It—And So Will You

Some people struggle with self esteem and doubt their ability to succeed; others have trouble motivating themselves to stick with a plan or get too obsessed with the number on the scales. No matter who you are, weight loss is a true emotional roller coaster, filled with confidence-boosting highs and demoralizing lows. I struggled with all of these issues. I rode this roller coaster—I had a front-row seat and often felt like my seat belt was going to rip off. When my weight loss stalled, I panicked. But I also knew that by exercising and eating well, I was giving my body its greatest chance of recovery and health and that this plateau wouldn't last forever. As you move from week to week you'll begin to develop and cultivate an arsenal of tools to combat discouraging feelings and push through. My clients have fantastic weeks, pretty good weeks, and average weeks. As far as I'm concerned there is never a bad week once you have decided to get in shape. From the day you make a real commitment your future shines brightly. After all, nobody—*nobody*—can remain overweight if they eat well, lift weights, and exercise regularly. *That* is reality.

How Soon Will You See Results?

By the end of Week 1: A decrease in joint and back pain. More sound sleep. Feel lighter. Reduction in waist size as you begin eating more manageable portions.

By the end of Month 1: Better mood. Easier time falling asleep and waking up. Clearer skin. Improved self-esteem.

By the end of Month 3: Friends will start telling you how great you look. You'll have more energy (no more of that 3 p.m. slump) and will notice yourself looking forward to your workouts.

By the end of Month 6: Most readers should be able to attain their goal within six months.

PJ's Pointer

Here is the single most important equation I've come up with:

Healthy eating + weights + cardio
+ self-belief =
body and mind transformation

When I began exercising again, I had less than zero confidence. It took me three weeks to motivate myself to complete a full workout finally, and I left it feeling miserable because I was still filling my body with unhealthy food. I didn't think the rules applied to me—I thought *I* could cut corners. But you can't expect to see results from exercise if you're not putting in the hard work with food. Once I got myself into a strong, three-pronged routine (healthy eating, cardio, weights), however, I saw real changes within the first week.

LOSE THAT, GAIN THIS

The magic number when it comes to weight loss is 10 percent—at least in the beginning.[3] Even if you have your sights set on a larger number, start with 10 percent. Breaking your goal up into smaller, more manageable chunks will make the journey seem less daunting. Furthermore, check out what else you have to gain just by losing 10 percent:

If You Lose 10 Percent, You Gain . . .
- Lower blood pressure, cholesterol, and blood sugar levels.[4]
- Decreased risk of Type 2 diabetes, a weight-related chronic condition in which your body can't make enough (or properly utilize) insulin, the hormone responsible for converting food to usable energy. Already diagnosed with Type 2 diabetes? Ditching 10 percent of your weight can improve your symptoms and prevent complications.[5]
- Significantly increased energy.
- *More* weight loss. Getting a 10 percent loss under your belt will really shore up your confidence for when you attempt the second 10 percent, which reminds me . . .
- A shopping trip for new clothes!

PJ's
Pointer

Far too often I see people attempt to lose massive amounts of weight by doing everything to the extreme, yet it never shows in their overall appearance. When you lose fat correctly through eating well, exercising, and lifting weights, you transform your body—and the changes in size and shape are amazing! Losing ten pounds doesn't really excite people, but dropping a pant size or a dress size as the result of a ten-pound loss motivates even the most pessimistic client to soldier on.

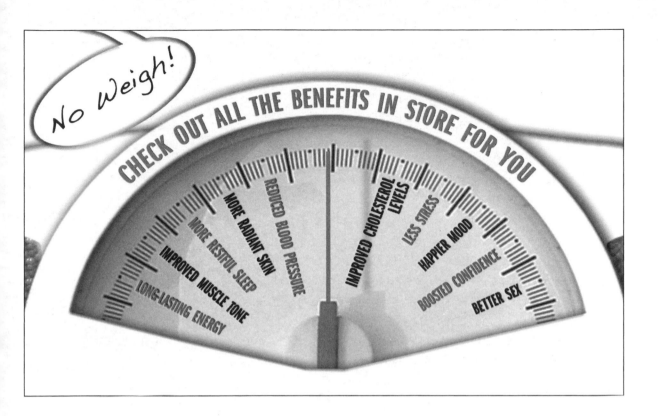

"Since losing the weight, my life has changed drastically. I recently celebrated—really cele-brated—my birthday for the first time in seven years. My driver's license had been expired for a decade because my seat belt didn't fit: I just renewed it. My blood pressure has drastically improved, and my sleep apnea disappeared. Now, when I look in the mirror, I smile."
—**Dora Dogas,** age thirty-five, lost 198 pounds . . . and counting

EXCESS BAGGAGE

How does too much weight hurt you? Let us count the ways. Compared to their thinner counterparts, overweight and obese people are more likely to:

- die early[6]
- die in a car accident[7]

- be depressed[8]
- have a heart attack or stroke[9]
- develop diabetes[10]
- be infertile—both men[11] and women[12]
- suffer from chronic pain[13]
- succumb to colon cancer[14]
- experience acid reflux[15]
- develop kidney stones[16]
- get addicted to drugs or alcohol[17]
- have heavy friends[18]

PJ's
Pointer

Imagine carrying a twenty-pound dumbbell around with you wherever you go. Heading off to work? Don't forget your dumbbell. Meeting friends for dinner? Grab that dumbbell. Heading upstairs to tuck your kids into bed? . . . You get my point. Now imagine how incredibly freeing it would feel to toss that weight in the garbage. *Everything* would be easier. That's how you'll feel when you lose your first 10 percent.

START SMART

Before beginning the KO-90 program consult your physician and make sure you're physically able to perform a range of exercises. Have him or her determine your baseline blood pressure and cholesterol. Most people, even if they're very overweight, can do *something*, even if it's just walking around the block.

Know Your Numbers

In addition to a full doctor's workup, you'll need to assess your beginning measurements and body-fat percentage. Record all of these measurements in your KO-90 Plan Journal in the back of the book (page 192).

Body-fat percentage. Many weight-loss plans emphasize your Body Mass Index, or BMI, a measure of body fat based on height and weight. The problem with BMI is that it can be terribly misleading, especially for men with more muscle mass. For example, George Clooney, at five-foot-eleven and an estimated 185 pounds, is technically overweight according to his BMI. At six-foot-two and 223 pounds, Dallas Cowboys' Tony Romo is nearly obese.

I typically use a pair of calipers to determine clients' body-fat percentage. Calipers look sort of like a cross between a compass and a pair of salad tongs and work by pulling skin and fat away from the muscle at multiple locations (I do a 7-point pinch test covering the chest, abdomen, thigh, tricep, axilla, subscapula, and suprailiac). Some gyms will offer alternate tools to measure body-fat percentage, such as handheld devices, which send a weak, pain-free electric signal through the body to measure composition. (Home body-fat scales work in the same manner.) But in my experience the results are often inaccurate. Pretty much any local gym or fitness center should have a pair of calipers on hand to measure your body-fat percentage.

The gold standard for body-fat testing is hydrostatic (underwater) weighing, in which a person is immersed in a large tank of water. The theory is that lean tissue will sink whereas fat will float, so an individual with more muscle will weigh more underwater than a person with a high percentage of body fat will. If you are interested in having your body-fat percentage tested by using this method and you live near a university, you could try contacting their physical therapy or athletic department, or you could visit www.bodyfattest.com to see if their mobile Get Tanked Mobile Lab will be in your neighborhood anytime soon. Once you have your initial results, record them in your KO-90 Plan Journal (page 192). Where do you fit in the following chart?

Body-Fat Percentage

LEVEL	WOMEN	MEN
Necessary to function	8–12%	3–5%
Athlete	13–19%	6–11%
Fitness	**20–25%**	**12–17%**
Average	26–31%	18–24%
Dangerous	32% +	25%+

Your goal is to reach that fitness sweet spot—20 to 25 percent for women and 12 to 17 percent for men. Anything above these figures veers into "average" territory. My job is to push you past "average." I want you to feel more than average; I want you to feel *fantastic*.

As I mentioned before, a loss of 1 to 2 percent of your body weight per week is an attainable goal. Attempting to drop more than that is unrealistic and will set you up for failure. Plus, you won't be losing fat—and you're not here to lose muscle, are you?

Body measurements. Using a fabric measuring tape, record the following measurements before starting and record them in your journal in the back of the book (page 192). You'll remeasure every month.

1. Chest—measure at the nipple line
2. Waist—measure smallest part of your torso, usually a few inches above your navel
3. Hips—measure at the widest part, usually around the hip bones
4. Thigh—measure the widest part, usually just beneath your glutes
5. Calves—measure at the widest part

Waist-to-hip ratio. Divide your waist measurement by your hip measurement for your waist-to-hip ratio. Record the figure in your journal in the back of the book (page 192). Again, you'll remeasure every month.

PJ's Pointer

Have you ever seen an overweight person at the gym, huffing and puffing as he bikes or stair-climbs as hard as he can? The reason he looks the same month after month is because he's *working out too hard*. Effective fat loss is achieved at 60 percent of your maximum heart rate. When you workout at top capacity and your heart rate skyrockets to 90 or even 100 percent, you're strengthening your heart, which is vital for circulation and cardiovascular fitness but fairly ineffective for fat loss. As you get fitter, incorporate "interval" training.

Target heart rate. To calculate your target heart rate, subtract your age from 220, then multiply by .60.

Age twenty-five: 220–25 = 195. 195 X .60 = 117 beats per minute
Age thirty-five: 220–35 = 185. 185 X .60 = 111 beats per minute
Age forty-five: 220–45 = 175. 175 X .60 = 105 beats per minute
Age fifty-five: 220–55 = 165. 165 X .60 = 99 beats per minute

Resting heart rate. Your resting heart rate, or RHR, is exactly what it sounds like: your heart rate at rest. The best time to find your resting heart rate is in the morning, after a good night's sleep and before you get out of bed.

For most people the heart beats about 60 to 80 times a minute while at rest. It rises during physical activity and lowers during a good night's sleep. Very physically fit people tend to have low RHRs—in fact, marathon runners can measure as low as 35 beats per minute! Unfortunately, overweight and obese individuals force their hearts to work extra hard simply to circulate blood, thereby straining the heart. When I reached my peak weight of 264 pounds, my heart rate was around 90, which was 50 percent higher and faster than when I began! It's now back to 60—evidence of a strong, efficient system.

To find your RHR, simply measure your pulse—at inner wrist or neck—for one minute. I've had clients with RHRs as high as 120, which is flat-out dangerous. With KO-90 you'll shoot for an ultimate RHR of around 60.

Maximum heart rate. To calculate your maximum heart rate, subtract your age from 220.

Age twenty-five: 220–25 = 195 beats per minute
Age thirty-five: 220–35 = 185 beats per minute
Age forty-five: 220–45 = 175 beats per minute
Age fifty-five: 220–55 = 165 beats per minute

Know your strength. To gauge your endurance and upper body, lower body, and core strength, grab a stopwatch with a minute hand and see how many push-ups and sit-ups you can perform in one minute. Then place your forearms on the floor and stretch out your legs in a "plank position" supporting yourself on your toes. Raise your torso off the floor, leaving only your toes and forearms grounded and see how many seconds you can hold this position. Then hop on an Elliptical machine at the gym and go as hard as you can for two minutes, checking to see what distance you've covered at the end as well as your heart rate. Mark these figures in your journal in the back of the book (page 192). Don't feel discouraged if you can barely eke out one push-up or get too winded to finish the two minutes on the cross-trainer; that just means you'll see progress even sooner. No one else needs to know your results—this is a competition only against yourself to be the healthiest, strongest person you can be. You'll repeat these tests on a monthly basis, monitoring your progress in your journal.

When I was heavy, I'd snack on donuts and chocolate bars—I'd even keep a family-size bag of Gummi Bears on me and pop them while training clients or driving. You know why? I was so exhausted from carrying around all that weight that I practically needed an IV supply of sugar to stay awake. Now that the weight is off, I snack on nuts and fruit—though Gummi Bears still have their time and place! The difference? I'm in control of my eating; my eating's not in control of me.

I know that working out in a gym can be incredibly intimidating, particularly when you're overweight. It seems like everyone there is thinner, fitter, and stronger than you are. But as someone who spends nearly half of his life in the gym, working and training, I can assure you that everyone there is so busy worrying about themselves that they barely have the time or energy to look at or judge you! Do not allow your fears to keep you at home or prevent you from testing your own strength. Before you know it, *you'll* be one of the lean, fit gym members inspiring *others* to get in shape.

Before, during, and after photos. There's nothing like a photograph to deliver raw, honest feedback about how you look. Have a friend you trust snap a front, side, and back shot of you. Then develop or download them (they won't do any good sitting in your camera) and paste them in your journal on page 191 or on your vision board. Repeat the process every month for a truthful visual documentation of your progress. Comparing monthly photos is far more effective than obsessing in the mirror every day. Changes in your body shape and size will be impossible to deny in these pictures, and their "Wow" factor will motivate you to soldier on.

SUCCESS STORY **BERNADETTE**

"While going to sleep at night and waking up in the morning, I would 'see' and 'feel' myself slim. I saw myself wearing specific outfits in smaller sizes and doing everyday things like supermarket shopping or going for a walk. I also visualized myself waking up and happily getting into gym gear and working out. This helped stop my negative thinking and enabled me to feel free and empowered."

—**Bernadette Clarebrough,** age fifty-one, lost 53 pounds

These pictures may be worth a thousand words, but I'll allow them to speak for themselves.

JANUARY 1, 2009

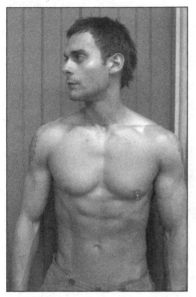 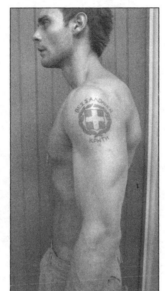 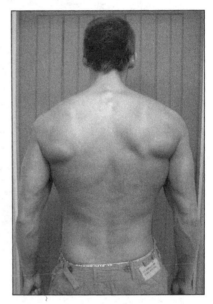

JULY 1, 2009

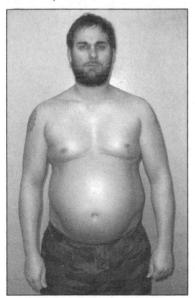 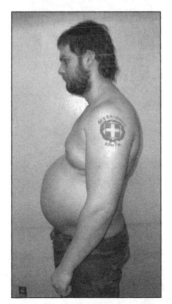 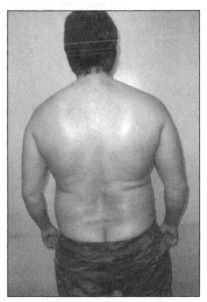

October 1, 2009

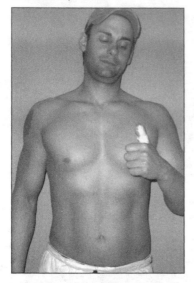
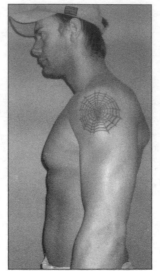
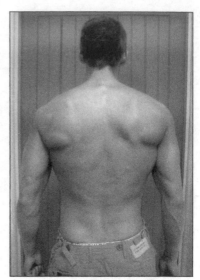

December 31, 2009

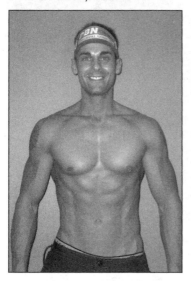
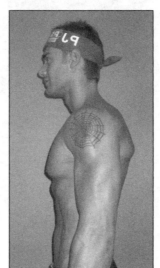
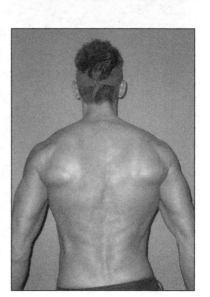

SUCCESS STORY **L I L Y**

"Most trainers have always been fit and healthy; they don't know what it's like to be over-weight, what it feels like when you go to a gym and are surrounded by people with great bodies. If you haven't walked in an overweight person's shoes, you will never truly know what it's like. PJ has been there and done that, both physically and emotionally."

—Lily Williams, age thirty-four, lost 33 pounds . . . and counting

PART 3

TAKE CHARGE

Psyching Yourself Up for a New Life

Typically, I'm not one to go around quoting Woody Allen, but he hit the nail on the head when he famously declared, "Half of life is showing up." All of my clients hear the same thing from me: "Showing up at the gym is half the battle. You just need to show up, and I'll take care of the rest." No, I don't complete the workouts for them, and I don't prepare meals for them. But I do teach them the steps they need to take and guide them through their journey.

By picking up this book, you have taken just as huge a step as if you were standing in the weight room with me right now. Making the decision to get fit is a challenging feat in and of itself; I know from experience that it would be far, far easier to maintain the status quo, eat what you want to eat, pretend the gym doesn't exist, and ignore the pleas of your physician, family, friends, or inner voice. But there comes a point when the pain of being unfit is so unbearable that you will do anything to change it.

During first meetings with clients it's not uncommon for them to utter self-defeating re-frains such as, "I'll never be able to lose fifty pounds—I can barely get rid of five," or "You're my last hope. If this doesn't work, I'm just going to be fat and miserable forever." If these sorts of thoughts have been hanging around in your mind, you need to banish them *right now*. Erase them off a mental chalkboard; write them down on a piece of paper and tear it up or set it on fire—do what you need to wipe your mental slate clean of negativity so you can start fresh. A bad attitude will only hamper your efforts, and this is a time when you need all of the glass-is-half-full thinking you can muster. If you continue to dwell on being overweight, think of exercise as torturous, or deem vegetables and grilled fish "rabbit food," you're setting yourself up for failure. My job is to set you up for success.

GETTING READY

Before you start exercising and changing your diet, you owe it to yourself to spend some time mentally preparing for the changes to come. Your success will depend in large part on how ready you are to tackle the challenges ahead. Losing weight is an intensive project, so think of this section of the book as your emotional weight-loss tool kit.

Make a List

Write down a list of reasons *why* you want to lose weight.* No motive is too big or too small. Read your list every day, keeping it nearby so you can pull it out during your most vulnerable moments (in the cab on your way to a foodie friend's party, after dinner when mindless snacking often attacks, or on the plane to visit your food-pusher parents). Some reasons to get you started:

> Why I Want To Lose Weight
> So I can climb the stairs without running out of breath
> So I can coach my kid's Little League team
> So I can look good in a form-fitting dress
> So I can avoid the heart disease that runs in my family
> So I can stop feeling embarrassed when people take pictures
> So my back doesn't hurt all the time
> So I can start shopping at mainstream clothing stores
> So I can feel strong
> So I can feel sexy
> So I will feel better about myself

*Create your own list on page 191.

Envision Yourself Thinner

I'm a huge believer in visualization. Your body can respond to thoughts and dreams as if they were actually happening. Need an example? Picture a packet of your favorite crisps. Inhale their smell; imagine the explosion of flavor as it hits your tongue. Are you salivating a little bit yet? Then I've made my point. Think crisps; taste crisps. Think thin; become thin.

I encourage you to find a picture of a person with your ideal body (keeping things realistic, of course) and post it somewhere conspicuous, like in your gym locker, on your refrigerator door, or even in the back of this book. The person may be an actor, singer, or even a past, slimmer version of yourself. One of my clients, Suzanne, weighed 171 pounds when we started. She scoured her favorite magazines and snipped out a few pictures of body types she thought were achievable. She kept a daily journal and posted the photos in it, along with her weekly weigh-ins. Suzanne currently weighs 138 pounds, just 10 pounds from her goal weight.

SUCCESS STORY **BERNADETTE**

"When I hit a plateau on the way, I began visualizing myself in certain clothes, seeing my stomach as toned and flat, and picturing myself moving through the world as a slim person. Driving my car and pushing the cart in the supermarket, I would visualize myself in a new, smaller pair of jeans and T-shirt. I also saw myself pulling fun, trendy new clothes out of my wardrobe and putting them on with an easy feeling before running out thc door."

—Bernadette Clarebrough, age fifty-one, lost 53 pounds

Later, I'll ask you to continue the visualization practices as you start working out. For me, picturing myself lifting weights and doing cardio on the Elliptical trainer, was crucial for psyching myself up to hit the gym again. It helped me recall how good I felt when I was healthy and active. Even if you've never belonged to a gym, dig into your past and find a memory you associate with feeling strong. Maybe it was when you were a child and playing at the park with friends. Or when you were involved in sports in high school.

Picture This **PJ's** Pointer

After six months of gluttony, motivating myself to start working out and eating right felt next to impossible. So I created a vision board. I taped a big sign to it that read, "80 KG: December 31, 2009" (that's in kilograms and is equal to 176 pounds). I also used an old modeling photo for my inspirational visualization pic. It reminded me what I was capable of achieving, and after six months of pushing myself and staying true to my goals I was able to reach that state once again and even surpass it.

KEEP IT OFF

Or when you taught your son how to ride a bike. If you've never exercised and are struggling with the visualization, then focus on your health as your motivation and picture yourself as you are right now. Take a good, hard look and ask yourself: Are you happy? If you're reading this book, I suspect the answer is no. Let's change that.

Know Thy Enemies

Trigger foods, emotional and binge eating, self-doubt, diet saboteurs, pressure from friends and family to eat or not eat—I had no real clue how many forces conspire against you when you're trying to lose weight until I took the journey myself. Now I have a clearer idea of what you're up against. It's critical that you know too.

WHAT'S YOUR TRIGGER?

First, identify your trigger foods and situations. Maybe you find turning down dessert impossible, no matter how gut-bustingly full you may feel from dinner. Or you can never stop at just one small handful of nuts—you keep plunging your hand back into the can for more and more. For some people heading out to see a movie triggers an almost Pavlovian response: "Must. Get. Popcorn." Figure out your triggers and then make a plan of attack for fighting back should they rear their ugly heads. If you arrive prepared, you're far more likely not to succumb.

ID EMOTIONAL EATING

On June 30, 2009, when I twisted my ankle while attempting to jog the day before my first workout, I was devastated—embarrassed, ashamed, depressed. And as you already know, I dealt with the uncomfortable emotions in a destructive way—by ordering pizza the following night. My pride stung just as badly as my ankle, and I knew that sinking my teeth into slice after slice of hot, melted cheese and pepperoni would make me feel a thousand times better (well, for ten minutes, anyway).

Head Triggers Off at the Pass

Trigger	Solution
The sweet smell of cookies	Avoid the baked goods aisle when grocery shopping. Wait outside while your friends stop at the bakery. Send your child off to school with birthday fruit cups instead of Snickerdoodles.
Enormous serving portions (e.g., tubs of ice cream, bulk sized bags of dried fruit, gigantic restaurant entrées)	Purchase single-serving sizes or divide bulk-container items into smaller plastic baggies. When dining out, automatically ask your server to reserve and box up half of your dish (bonus: instant leftovers for tomorrow!).
Buttery, salty movie theater popcorn	Smuggle in your own air-popped popcorn from home. After all, you wouldn't eat three McDonald's Quarter Pounders topped with a dozen pats of butter while catching a flick, would you? A medium movie popcorn and soda combo has the same number of calories and saturated fat (1610 and 60, respectively).*
Family meals	Prepare a healthy dish at home—with enough to share—and bring it with you to the event. Don't arrive famished. Pile your plate high with salad and veggies (skipping anything creamed, fried, or glistening in oil), using meat and poultry as side dishes.
Cooking	Pop some sugar-free gum in your mouth or sip on herbal tea to keep your mouth occupied to avoid sneaking bites of brownie batter or rice casserole while baking or cooking—those nibbles contain calories (two spoonfuls of cookie dough can total 500 calories!**).
Leftover food on your plate	Place your napkin over the plate, ask the server to take it away, or even sprinkle pepper on it to discourage wasteful noshing. Don't fall victim to the "I don't want to waste food" mentality; if you eat when you're not hungry, you're still wasting it—only it will end up as excess fat rather than in the garbage can.

*"Two Thumbs Down' for Movie Theater Popcorn," Center for Science in the Public Interest, November 18, 2009, http://www.cspinet.org/new/200911182.html.
**Leslie Goldman, "Eat, Drink, and Still Shrink," *Women's Health*, December 2010, http://www.womenshealthmag.com/weight-loss/healthy-eating-plan.

Emotional eating happens to the best of us, wreaking havoc by causing us to use food as a security blanket. It fills us when we feel empty. It soothes us when we're in pain. It occupies us when we're bored. It distracts us from unpleasant feelings—immersing your senses in a gooey pizza pie is far easier than focusing on the (very real) fear that your eating is endangering your health. And we never reach for steamed broccoli or a tuna sandwich, but rather creamy chocolate, greasy potato chips, or French fries dipped in melted cheese. No one emotionally eats a salad.

Unfortunately, the immediate relief we experience from those sugary, fatty, salty goodies is fleeting, and we're left feeling even worse than we did when we started. Because now, on top of dealing with the anger, fear, or shame that drove us to eat in the first place, we must face the fact that we just self-sabotaged with unnecessary calories, fat, and sodium. That knowledge only intensifies the negative emotions, and a wicked cycle ensues. Adding insult to injury, overweight individuals are more likely than underweight people are to eat in response to negative moods and situations.[3]

I would estimate that the vast majority of my clients struggle with emotional eating. About 75 percent of them will overeat in an effort to deal with stress; the remaining 25 percent will actually restrict themselves. That latter strategy might sound smart, but starving their bodies slows their metabolism and sets them up for binge eating. Plus, they show up for sessions with zero energy.

Everyone has different reasons for emotional eating, but common culprits include work stress, financial strain, health concerns, relationship problems, unemployment, fatigue, and even bad weather. (There's a form of depression called Seasonal Affective Disorder that is characterized by irritability, extreme fatigue, withdrawal from social activities, increased appetite, and carbohydrate cravings.) With a little knowledge of biology, this all makes perfect sense. When you're depressed, your levels of serotonin—the feel-good brain chemical—plummet. In response, you crave high-carb foods, which naturally enhance serotonin production. Chips, fries, and cake essentially act like edible Prozac, soothing and comforting you after a fight with your partner or a lousy day at work.[4]

Check Yourself before You Wreck Yourself

I once heard a trainer tell a client to ask herself the following question whenever she found herself mindlessly wandering into the kitchen: "Could I eat a big salad with grilled fish on top right now?" If the answer is "No," he said, then she wasn't truly hungry and was eating for comfort. The next time you find yourself automatically reaching for chips or ice cream, give yourself a reality check. Are you bored? Lonely? Anxious? Sad? If the act of recognizing your emotional eating isn't enough to deter you, try writing it down in a journal or the back of this book. In fact, keeping track of your snacks and meals is a great idea. Try it for a week, using the pages in your health journal at the back of the book. Keep track of your snacks and meals, noting what you eat as well as recording the main emotion you felt at the time and ranking your hunger on a scale of one to ten. After just a few days a telling pattern should emerge.

Drink a Tall Glass of Water

Mistaking thirst for hunger is not uncommon. If you feel hungry, drink eight ounces of water and wait twenty minutes to see if the cravings have passed. This takes discipline, but once you've tried it a few times it gets easier, and in the meantime you might get so immersed in a new activity that your emotional eating gets derailed.

Craft a New Comfort Strategy

Figure out a way to deal with your emotions that doesn't involve eating. Here are some alternatives:

Head outside for some fresh air and take a long walk.
Call a friend and vent.
Grab a book or newspaper and head out to a nearby café for a cup of tea.
Occupy your hands with a project like knitting or drawing.
Occupy your mind with a crossword or Sudoku puzzle.
Do the laundry.
Play with your dog.
Give yourself a mani pedi.
Take a fifteen-minute nap.

SHOW ME THE SCIENCE

Do You Need a Brownie . . . or a Hug?

When researchers at the Cornell Food and Brand Lab asked 1,004 Americans why they indulge in their favorite comfort food, 86 percent said they ate when they were happy, 74 percent when they wanted to reward themselves, 39 percent when they were depressed or lonely.[5]

BINGE EATING

Binge Eating Disorder is America's best-kept secret, affecting a staggering number of people—more than anorexia and bulimia *combined*.[6] We've all had the experience of indulging in far more food than we really needed, but for sufferers of BED, overeating accompanied by a sense of being out of control can be an everyday experience. People with BED typically eat rapidly during a binge, eat until they're uncomfortably full, eat alone due to embarrassment over the amount of food they're consuming, and suffer feelings of disgust, depression, or guilt as a result.[7]

Stress, depression, and dieting are all common binge triggers, and the consequences of long-term bingeing include high blood pressure, Type 2 diabetes, heart disease, GI issues, joint pain, and all of the other ramifications of obesity. Unfortunately, our society stigmatizes binge eaters in a way that people with eating disorders like anorexia or bulimia are not: bingers are viewed as gluttonous and lacking willpower, whereas anorexics and bulimics are often treated very gingerly and generally not criticized in an open and direct fashion by others. But eating disorders—of any kind—are physically damaging and emotionally destructive. If you think you have a problem with BED, I urge you to seek help. Contact the National Association of Anorexia Nervosa and Associated Disorders at www.anad.org or Overeaters Anonymous at www.oa.org.

FINDING FAULT FOR OUR FAT

In January of 2011 Starbucks rolled out a new size category of drink called the Trenta. Weighing in at thirty-one ounces, the Trenta is actually larger than the average adult human's stomach capacity.[8]

In a society in which we are encouraged to consume literally gut-busting proportions, is it any wonder so many of us are overweight? I'm not saying we can place 100 percent of our waistline blame on Starbucks's shoulders, but the fact is that we live in an obesogenic world, where practically everything around us pushes us closer and closer toward obesity. Researcher James O. Hill, PhD, of the University of Colorado, calls obesity "a normal response to the American environment."[9] And former Food and Drug Administration chief David Kessler, MD, estimates that up to seventy million of us have some degree of conditioned hyper-eating, meaning our eating is excessive and driven by motivational forces that we find difficult to control. Those factors include:

- *Biology.* Marketing-savvy food producers have tapped into consumer preferences for fat, salt, and sugar, pumping our cuisine full of ingredients that are devoid of nutrition. Not only that, fat and sugar have legitimate addictive capabilities: a 2010 study in *Nature Neuroscience* confirmed that, in animals, fast food affects the brain in a similar way to cocaine or heroin.[10] The pleasure centers of the brain become so overstimulated that more and more food is required just to feel normal.
- *Portions.* Restaurant portions, snack-food sizes, and plate diameters have mushroomed in the past few decades, and research consistently shows that the more food we are offered or the bigger our plates, the more we eat, regardless of how hungry we are or how much we like the food. In one study moviegoers eating popcorn out of supersized buckets consumed 49 percent more than those served from medium-sized bags, despite the fact that they had claimed not to like the taste.[11]
- *Modern technology.* Computers, video games, and high-definition TV encourage increasingly sedentary lifestyles. Add to that the fact that, with the exception of a few major cities, driving is the norm—even to the corner market or gym—and we're moving less than ever before.

To say you're up against a lot is a wild understatement. Although changes are being enacted to combat America's obesogenic environment—many restaurants are now required to post calorie counts and First Lady Michelle Obama is tackling childhood obesity with her "Let's Move" campaign—the fact remains that weight loss can be extraordinarily challenging when you're surrounded by oversized portions and addictive snacks. That's why sticking to the guidelines I give you in KO-90 is imperative. By drastically limiting the amount of fat, sugar, and salt, you'll help train your taste buds and mind to adapt to more natural-tasting foods, and you will find your junk-food cravings actually dissipating. I know it sounds crazy right now, but it's incredible how delicious a sweet potato can taste after a week without candy and ice cream.

I'll also be encouraging you to fit in short bouts of exercise whenever you can. That means running an errand on foot instead of taking the car, hand delivering a message to a coworker instead of e-mailing it, or forgoing the elevator for the stairs. Instead of plopping down on the couch after dinner and zoning out in front of the television, walk around the block a few times. Take your dog—or a neighbor's dog—out on a hike. Park in the far corner of the lot when shopping, thereby forcing yourself to cover just a little more ground to reach your destination. You'll find that building in mini-sessions of activities grows easier with time until it becomes second nature.

DEFEND YOURSELF AGAINST DIET SABOTAGE

This is going to sound harsh, but the people closest to you are often your worst enemies when it comes to losing weight. Diet saboteurs are everywhere, lurking in the bodies of your closest friends, your parents and in-laws, your spouse or partner. They say things like, "We love you just the way you are" or "You get so cranky when you're dieting" or "You're looking too skinny." I have one client who had a solid fifty pounds to lose. Once she shed the first five, her friends started telling her to stop, that she looked great and was taking it too far.

That's not a real friend. Your support system should do just that: support you in your endeavor to become healthy. What happens, though, is that they get nervous. They might start to wonder, "Well, if *she's* starting to exercise, maybe *I* need to as well." Attempting to thwart your efforts is a lot easier than making real changes for themselves.

In the case of a family member, your mother might constantly try to force-feed you, even if you have asked her to stop. Chalk her actions up to a pervasive "food equals love" mentality. If your partner is the one sabotaging you, he might be nervous that once you trim down, the opposite sex will notice you more and so you might be tempted to stray.

Before you start kicking these people out of your life, understand that their thoughts are likely operating on a subconscious level. They don't *want* you to be out of shape. They don't *want* you to have high blood pressure and an increased risk of a heart attack. They're just improperly interpreting your get-healthy efforts as an attack on their own unhealthy lifestyle or as a rejection of their love.

SUCCESS STORY **BERNADETTE**

"My coworkers tell me I should 'enjoy my life' and eat the treats they keep bringing around. I don't say things like 'Oh, I'd better not' or 'I want to, but I'm on a diet.' Instead, I tell them 'The choice between being healthy and not having diabetes and eating X, Y, Z is pretty easy,' or 'I'm happy with my salad, thanks.'"

—**Bernadette Clarebrough,** age fifty-one, lost 53 pounds

One way to head diet sabotage off is to stay quiet about your weight-loss plan—at least in the beginning. Some experts suggest telling everyone about your goals to build accountability, but I've found that doing so is like holding up a giant neon sign that reads, "Sabotage me!" There's no need to sit down to a meal and announce, "No mac and cheese for me tonight—I'M ON A DIET!" Instead, try the following approaches:

Saboteur City

The saboteur	What they say	Your response
Your spouse	"You're no fun to be around when you're dieting" or "Look, honey, I brought you home pizza—your favorite!"	"I don't get it—yesterday you told me you were happy that I was getting healthy, but today you're bringing home pizza" or "I'm not trying to force you to lose weight, but this is something I need to do for myself, and I need you to be supportive . . . or at least keep the pizza out of the house!"
Your friends	"Oh, come on, live a little! Just have some fries with us! Quit being such a Goody Two-shoes."	"You guys, I would love to, but you know how much my plan means to me. I could really use your support right now." Or instead of going to dinner, invite your friends on a more active date, like a long walk or bike ride.
Your mother	"I spent all day cooking your favorite meatloaf . . . and you're not even going to have one bite?!"	"Mom, you know I love you—and your meatloaf—but I'm trying to make some healthy changes in my life. Maybe next time you could make your famous [insert healthy dish here]—I'd love to dig into that!"

SHOW ME THE SCIENCE

Are Your Friends Making You Fat?

A 2007 *New England Journal of Medicine* study found that having an overweight friend makes you 57 percent more likely to be overweight yourself. Having an obese spouse raises your odds by 37 percent.[13]

Arm Yourself

Now that you've identified the multiple sources conspiring against you and your get-fit plan, it's time to prepare yourself for a hearty defense. These tools will help keep you motivated, inspired, and empowered, so when you do find yourself having dinner with a sabotaging coworker at a restaurant that calls a pound of pasta "dinner" or are dreading hitting the gym because it's dark and rainy outside and you just want to curl up with a bag of bagel chips, you can push on through to the other side.

BUDDY UP

There's power in numbers! Working out with a friend is a fantastic motivator because it forces you to be accountable to someone other than yourself. Ditching the gym is easy if nobody is expecting you—not so much when you know your buddy is waiting for you at 6 a.m. for a fifteen-minute Elliptical session. I wish I'd had a partner to get fit with, but I chose to go it alone because I was trying to make the journey as difficult as possible (part of my experiment involved pushing myself to my absolute limits). But a University of Pittsburgh study found that dieters who had one other person check in on them lost twice as much weight as those who didn't. If you can't get a friend to join in, ask a coworker. Invite your partner on an active date, or find an online support group. You can even tweet your gym visits on Twitter as a way to stay accountable: once you type, "Off to Spin class," you'll feel obligated to go, and announcing "Just walked three miles!" will net you words of encouragement from friends. And try finding a weight-loss mentor—someone you respect who has lost weight and kept it off for an extended period of time. Tap them for advice, inspiration, and fitness and eating tips along the way.

BUST THROUGH PLATEAUS

I'd estimate that a weight-loss plateau sidelines 99 percent of my clients at least once. Plateaus occur when your metabolism starts to slow as the result of lean-tissue loss. In the beginning stages of weight loss the weight might seem to fall off of you as your body burns stored energy for fuel. But there comes a point, usually around month three or four, when you need to eat less and/or move more to get the scales to budge. Plateaus are incredibly frustrating, but take comfort in the knowledge that they are also common.

When you find this type of obstacle confronting you, I encourage you really to think about your routine. I find that most plateaus occur because of excessive cardio or a lack

Three months after I started trying to shed the weight my scales seemed to stop moving. The stall in progress was seriously challenging for me, and I felt lost as to how I would turn it around. At that point I hadn't truly committed to cardio because I wanted to prove that it was possible to get fit by just eating correctly. Clearly, that plan was backfiring. Plus, I had this twisted idea that I was different—that because I'd been so fit before, different rules applied to me. I realized that weekly weigh-ins and early-morning cardio were two crucial elements missing from my plan. I needed to build both self-awareness and self-esteem. Once I changed things up and integrated these principles, the weight started coming off again.

of sleep. My clients often inadvertently complicate things for themselves, especially after the halfway point of their weight loss, as they pile on cardio work without consulting with me in an effort to speed up the process. But excessive hours of running or Spinning combined with a calorie deficit will cause your body to "freak out" as it enters starvation mode, slowing your metabolism to protect itself. Furthermore, you'll be exhausted and may even start to feel depressed and agitated when you don't see the results you're working so diligently for. Matters can quickly spiral downward from there, as your body stores extra fat calories as it prepares for the upcoming famine.

There will be some weeks when you appear to have lost very little—or even no—weight. But that doesn't mean your body isn't still changing internally. Muscles are growing, fat stores are diminishing, self-confidence is growing. I always tell my clients: weight loss isn't the only goal. Looser-fitting clothes, an uplifted mood, and compliments from other people are better indicators of your progress. There's no simple recipe for fat loss, and no eating or exercise routine guarantees you will shed half a pound every day, seven days a week. You might drop four pounds one week and only one pound the next. The good news is that you *can* and *will* bust through this plateau. Make sure you do the following:

RE-EXAMINE YOUR HABITS

Be honest with yourself: Are you sticking to your nutrition plan and hitting the gym as often as you should? Often, as clients lose a significant amount of weight in the beginning, they subconsciously loosen some of the rules, like dipping into the bread basket while dining out or indulging in an after-work cocktail or two. But little slips here and there quickly add up.

REDEDICATE YOURSELF

Get back into the swing of things by recommitting yourself to your end goal. If you've stopped your visualization exercises, pick up where you left off. Make sure you're not skipping breakfast or snacks in an effort to save calories. Integrate more nongym activity into your day, like hopping off the train a stop early and walking, doing lunges as you clean up around the house, or getting up to change the channel on the TV instead of using the remote control.

MIX THINGS UP

It is said that the definition of insanity is doing the same thing over and over and expecting different results. The body's in-built memory needs to be shaken up to keep it from growing too lazy. Sometimes, all it takes is a change in eating or exercise routine. Tweak your meals, eat at slightly different times, incorporate new machines or different walking paces, or change your weight workouts. As you grow more familiar with your gym you'll learn your way around the various pieces of equipment and will almost instantly recognize which machines or free-weight exercises are for which muscle group. This way, you can spice things up, confuse your body with fresh exercises, and smash through that plateau!

STAY MOTIVATED

A dip in motivation can quickly cause your results to backslide. The mind rules the body and can seriously impact your success in a positive or negative way. Remind yourself of your overall goal or goals (maybe pull out the list of reasons you wrote on page 191). Acknowledge all of your success to remind yourself of where you started. I find that a lack of motivation is often the result of frustration, to which I say this: even if it takes you a year to get in shape and be healthy and happy, it is *only one year*. One year is miniscule in comparison to the years spent putting on weight and a potential lifetime of feeling miserable. And the reality is that most people won't require a year to reach their goal; six months is usually sufficient. If you have fifty pounds to lose, break it down into manageable sections and take it ten pounds at a time. Eating clean, lifting weights, and doing cardio before breakfast (more on this in Parts 4 and 5) are the fastest, most effective methods to get in shape, no matter how big you are at the starting line. Lapsing into moments of frustration and even apathy along the way is normal. But keep your eyes on the final prize—whether that's a smaller pair of pants, running a charity 5K, or drop-

After getting caught with those two pizzas following my inaugural July 1 workout, I used it as an excuse to continue stuffing my face. The next morning I had bacon and eggs on buttered toast for breakfast. What I *should* have done was recognize my blunder, wipe the pepperoni grease from my hands, and start fresh with a cup of oatmeal spiked with cinnamon. Mistakes happen. *Life* happens. Don't let a little slip-up balloon into a bender. Follow this Golden Rule: don't try to fix the past; instead, look to the future.

ping your cholesterol level thirty points—and remember that people are rooting for you: your family, your friends, and me.

FORGIVE YOURSELF IF YOU MESS UP

You slipped up and ate a cheeseburger and fries? You ditched the gym two days in a row? The world is not going to end. One bad meal will not derail your efforts. What *will* get you into trouble is allowing that unhealthy dinner or skipped weightlifting session to mushroom into a bingeing bender or days of total inactivity. All too often, we tear ourselves down for making a mistake and say, "To hell with it!" and then allow an all-or-nothing mentality to lead us down a path of destruction. Rather than berate yourself, wipe the slate clean and reflect on the progress you *have* made. Thinking about your achievements will help you deal with momentary failures, turning those failures into learning opportunities. Soon enough you'll start to see an upward trend of success. You'll make mistakes, but you shouldn't make the same mistake twice.

CATCH SOME ZZZs

"Lose weight while you sleep!" sounds like an overhyped infomercial claim, but the truth is that logging quality sleep will set you up for successful fat loss. That's because sleep is a critical regulator of body weight and metabolism. Two hunger-regulating hormones,

SHOW ME THE SCIENCE
Sleep Less, Weigh More
Researchers at Stanford University and University of Wisconsin found that volunteers who clocked less than eight hours a night had higher body-fat percentages than those who logged more sleep, and those who slept the least weighed the most.[14]

leptin and ghrelin, govern appetite. Ghrelin stimulates appetite, and leptin tells your brain when you're full. When you skimp on sleep, your leptin levels plummet, rendering your stomach an endless pit. Poor sleep also drives ghrelin levels up, juicing your appetite. Just a few nights of tossing and turning can weaken your resolve to choose the turkey on whole wheat over the sausage calzone. By making sleep a priority, you'll have an infinitely easier time making healthy eating decisions.

WHEN TO SEEK OUTSIDE HELP

Many of my clients view me as their therapist, and it's a role I'm honored to fill. They confide in me, showing me their weaknesses and strengths. In return, I encourage and empower them. I never judge. The feeling of being criticized for being overweight is still fresh in my mind, so I know that lack of willpower, laziness, or any of the other fallacies surrounding obesity are simply not true.

That said, if you are struggling with depression, binge eating, or a sense of hopelessness, you need to seek out a mental health professional for counseling. If you get yourself on track emotionally, you'll have a much easier time embarking on the weight-loss journey.

You'll also find that simply making the decision to get healthy and then taking steps to achieve that goal will help lift the fog of depression. When I was obese, I walked around like a miserable sack of potatoes. My poor mood severely impacted those close to me—my friends, my clients, my girlfriend. But as soon as I started losing weight—even just a few pounds—my mood lifted. I found myself talking more, joking around with friends, and being more affectionate with Lisa. After I'd hit the thirty-pound mark, I started socializing a lot more, attending parties, and shopping for new clothes. You'll find that even the smallest change can bring about boatloads of confidence.

PART 4

GET THE JUNK OUT

Fuel Your Body

Ready to jump in? Fantastic. As I explained, the numbers 60/30/10 will guide you for the next twelve weeks. That's the scientifically proven ratio of protein to carbohydrates to fat that will allow you to shed fat, build muscle, gain energy, and achieve the life you want. It's the combination I myself followed to return to my pre-obese size. It's likely drastically different from what you're used to eating, but this is a change worth fighting for. Believe me—I know that the types and preparations of food in my plan can seem intimidating and even strict. But the truth is that your stomach and mind will quickly acclimate to your revamped nutrition plan, and you'll find that food simply tastes better and more satisfying when prepared simply and wholesomely. As you cut sugary, salty, and fatty garbage out of your meal plan, your taste buds will not only adapt but also sharpen. Fueling yourself with clean, natural foods will just flat-out feel *awesome*, and that will motivate you to keep going. Plus, you can look forward to a slightly more relaxed version after three months, with a few of your favorite indulgences returning for cameo appearances.

First, you'll need to re-educate yourself on exactly what healthy eating is. You wouldn't believe how many clients come to me, thinking they're choosing healthy foods, yet their meals include salad drenched in dressing and sprinkled with cheese; pasta with Bolognese sauce; vegetables cooked in butter, oil, and salt; or homemade pizzas topped with processed meats. Other hidden saboteurs include

Fight Back — PJ's Pointer

Dedicate time, emotions, and effort to working on your relationship with food. You wouldn't stay with someone who abused you, would you? Junk-food addiction is a form of self-abuse.

anything with the word "diet" or "lite" in it. Although these packaged items may seem like healthy choices, they're often packed with sugar and salt to compensate for the missing fat and have been processed to a point where the ingredients are beyond recognition.

The KO-90 plan banks heavily on lean protein, produce, and whole grains. As you progress, you'll be able to add in a few more carbs, including fruit. Let's get started by taking a look at the key principles of KO-90 in greater depth.

EAT BREAKFAST

Let's say you finish dinner at 8 p.m., fall asleep around 10 p.m., and wake up at 6 a.m. That's ten hours that your body is humming along without food. So many people slap the snooze button a few times, roll out of bed and into the shower, and then race off to work with nothing in their belly but high-octane coffee. By the time they arrive at the office at 8 a.m., it's been twelve hours—an entire *half-day*—since their body has received any nutrition. At around 10 a.m., a coworker brings in a sugary coffee cake drizzled with icing and laced with pecans. I ask you, what on earth is going to be able to stop anyone from lunging at that dessert (it's not really a breakfast) as if it's the last thing on earth?

I'll tell you what would stop them: a hearty breakfast. The more nutritious your first meal is, the less likely you are to crave junk throughout the day. According to the National Weight Control Registry (NWCR), a group of six thousand–plus people who have lost significant amounts of weight and kept it off for long periods of time, eating breakfast is a critical component to sustained weight loss. In fact, an impressive 78 percent of NWCR members eat breakfast every day, as they find it helps curb hunger and overeating later in the afternoon and evening.[1] Breakfast was an essential part of my day as I was losing the weight, and it continues to be today. But *when* you eat can be just as important as *what* you eat. With KO-90 I want you to hold off just a bit on eating and get your cardio in first. Morning workouts should always be done first thing in the morning on an empty stomach. It's called "fasted training," and it helps you by forcing your body to turn fat reserves—rather than the cereal you just ate for breakfast—into fuel.

A solid breakfast might be a veggie egg-white omelet, or oatmeal and a no-carb protein shake, or poached eggs and steamed spinach with a side of grilled asparagus. For more ideas and recipes, turn to the Meal Plan section beginning on page 57.

EAT CLEAN

As we discussed in the previous chapter, continuous clean eating lays at the heart of the KO-90 plan. Clean eating is exactly what it sounds like: food that hasn't been processed, that is as close to its natural state as possible. You'll be enjoying whole, natural foods that don't come with a label or wrapper (except maybe some paper packaging from the fish counter). Fresh and frozen produce, lean meats, and whole grains will be your body's friends. Further, part of eating clean means drastically re-

ducing your intake of sugar, salt, and fat. Sugar is high in mostly empty calories, offering little to no nutritional value. It worsens your cholesterol, rots your teeth, and promotes obesity, thus putting you at risk for a slew of chronic conditions, including heart disease and diabetes. (Fruit does supply cancer-fighting antioxidants and fiber, but unfortunately, it's also quite high in sugar and throws off the 60/30/10 balance. Once you near your goal weight, fruit is one of the very first items you'll add back into your diet.) "Clean" carbohydrates, like sweet potatoes, oatmeal, and long-grain white rice, will keep your blood-sugar level on an even keel, powering you through workouts without causing midafternoon energy slumps. So wave goodbye to breads and pastas as well as sugary drinks

SUCCESS STORY **SUZANNE**

"When it comes to eating clean, it gets easier and easier because I see results on a weekly basis. It is amazing to see such change in my body—and the effect it has on my mental well-being."

—**Suzanne Konstantinides,** age forty-six, lost 33 pounds . . . and counting

like juices, soda, fat-bomb coffeehouse concoctions, Red Bull, and sports drinks. I don't even want you drinking diet soda; besides causing bloating and gassiness, research shows it can spike appetite, thereby fueling weight *gain*, not loss.[2] You may think those things will help you get healthy, but in fact it's the exact opposite.

Low in Fat

KO-90 is low in fat as well. Butter will be evicted from your refrigerator. Cheese is no longer welcome at the dinner table. It's time to learn how to enjoy vegetables that

Omega-3 fatty acids are a major buzzword in the health and nutrition fields, and with excellent reason. These heart-healthy fats—found primarily in fatty fish such as salmon and sardines as well as walnuts, flaxseeds, and soybeans (and a slew of new products including peanut butter and milk are now being fortified)—have been repeatedly shown to help reduce the risk of everything from heart disease and stroke to joint pain, depression, and even certain skin conditions. The secret behind their power: anti-inflammatory properties that help control inflammation in the heart, brain, tissues, and joints.

Although the first three months of KO-90 have you enjoying white fish, once you reach the maintenance phase, I encourage you to start adding in salmon and sardines (if you appreciate the taste, of course!). In the meantime I'll ask you to supplement your meals with flaxseed oil (a half teaspoon, or two liquid capsules, three times a day). Flaxseed oil is a rich source of an essential fatty acid called alpha-linolenic acid, a biologic precursor to omega-3 fatty acids. If you'd rather eat your fatty acids than swallow them in pill form, try mixing a half teaspoon with some balsamic vinegar and pouring it over a salad for a warm, nutty flavor infusion.

haven't been dipped in batter and deep-fried in oil. The saturated fat found in pork, marbled red meat, cheese, and other high-fat dairy sticks around for a long time after being swallowed, plugging up your arteries and hiking your risk of heart disease, Type 2 diabetes, and cancer, not to mention padding your belly and thighs with a blanket of flab. Small amounts of healthy fats, like flaxseed oil and omega 3s, are included in the plan, but I do not encourage large quantities, like that found in a piece of salmon or half an avocado or a large handful of nuts. When you're targeting fat loss, taking in large amounts of fat—no matter how "good" they may be—will not help your cause. Once you've reached your goal weight, you'll be able to add back in nuts and other healthy fats. To ensure you are receiving adequate fats, I recommend a half-teaspoon of flaxseed oil (or two liquid capsules) three times a day. Alternatively, you can drizzle a half-teaspoon over your salad along with balsamic vinegar. That way you still get the health benefits of the oil, but you're in total control of the amount.

Low in Salt

Salt gets the boot too. Although fat and sugar attract a lot of attention, I consider salt the world's next giant killer. People tend to overlook sodium, not realizing how much of it can be found in soups, frozen dinners, prepackaged and processed foods, fast food—it's even in bread and cheese! The US government recently released the revised 2010 Dietary Guidelines for Americans. Chief among the recommendations: reduce daily sodium intake to less than 2,300 milligrams (mg). (Those age fifty-one and older, African American of any age, or anyone who has hypertension, diabetes, or chronic kidney disease—about half of the US population, including children, and the majority of adults—should slash sodium to 1,500 mg.)[3] The problem: salt is in everything, from more obvious sources like chips and hamburgers to more surprising sources like cottage cheese (459 mg per 4-ounce serving) and Raisin Bran (350 mg per cup). A single can of Campbell's Chunky Old Fashioned Vegetable Beef Soup packs in 1,780 mg; even though the label might say 890 mg, the serving size is half a can, not one full can. Besides upping your risk for heart disease and stroke, sodium will derail your fat-loss efforts by hanging on to water and bloating you out.

Kids are the big losers because by the time they are able to make their own decisions, many are already addicted to sodium, having consumed it at such high levels for years. Families sitting down for a home-cooked dinner every evening seem to be a thing of the past, with more and more parents working longer hours and struggling to balance work commitments together with home life. As a result, many parents settle for take-out, fast food, or prepackaged dinners—all of which are spiked with sodium.

The majority of salt we consume every day comes from these types of processed foods, not from the salt shaker, so eating clean is the ideal way to reduce sodium intake and help ensure a far healthier life for your family. One effective way to limit salt is to replace it with a selection of tasty spices and herbs. Later in this chapter I'll introduce you to a whole rainbow of salt-free spices that can wake up your palate without trashing your arteries and abs.

Trust me when I say that you will be amazed at how fresh and pure food can taste when it hasn't been gunked up with fatty sauces or coated in a sea-salt crust. Think of how simply delicious a Honeycrisp apple can taste in September, with the juice rushing out as you take a big bite. All food has that flavor potential when cooked in a simple, healthy way, accented by herbs, spices, vinegars, or citrus juices. My clients are so used to masking foods' flavor with salt, fat, and sugar; they aren't addicted to the hamburger but rather the *fat* and *salt* in the hamburger. When you eat clean, you taste food for what it is.

"Just a Little" Can Add Up to a Lot PJ's Pointer

You can try to convince yourself that having "just one" mozzarella stick or "a little bite" of cake or "just a can" of soda won't be enough to derail your efforts. You'd be wrong. Allowing yourself multiple "little" cheats throughout the day will add up to *a lot* of trouble. You can easily rack up hundreds of extra calories, thereby sabotaging your work in the gym and at meals.

Pile on the vegetables. There's not much that vegetables *don't* do: their vitamins, minerals, and antioxidants help protect you from chronic illnesses such as heart disease, stroke, and cancer. Produce injects your body with energy-pumping iron and bone-building calcium, and its fiber keeps your digestive track moving along smoothly and promotes a feeling of satisfaction, filling you up for relatively few calories.

In general, you'll want to choose vibrant, deeply hued vegetables like spinach, peppers, eggplant, beets, and broccoli over their paler counterparts, such as iceberg lettuce: The intense color signifies a high concentration of antioxidants. You don't have to sit down to salad after salad after salad (although, if prepared properly, salads are an excellent option). Try substituting some spinach, mushrooms, or onions for the cheese in your egg-white omelet. Layer cucumbers and bell pepper slices with thinly sliced meat and roll them up for a quick snack. Make sure the majority of your plate is covered with vegetables, followed by lean protein and good-for-you carbs. And when you do have a salad, resist the temptation to douse it in blah-tasting fat-free salad dressing. Vitamins E and K, crucial for a healthy immune system and blood clotting, respectively, are fat-soluble, meaning they need to be eaten with a little fat to really do their job. So drizzle on a small amount of flaxseed oil with a few hearty splashes of balsamic vinegar for a tangy, satisfying, clean-eating dressing. Want something a bit warmer? Steaming veggies and topping with lemon juice, herbs, and vinegar is another one of my favorite ways to get my Rock Star Produce (see below) into my daily diet in a tasty, satisfying way.

Rock Star Produce

Become friends with the following veggies—they're all low in calories and sugar but high in volume, meaning you can fill yourself up without filling out. They're also packed with vitamins and water, helping you meet your daily nutrient and hydration needs without even trying.

Asparagus	Cucumber	Mushrooms
Bell peppers	Eggplant	Onions
Bok choy	Green beans	Radishes
Broccoli	Jicama	Spaghetti squash
Brussels sprouts	Kale	Spinach
Cauliflower	Lettuce (romaine, mixed	Swiss chard
Celery	greens, butter)	Tomatoes

Fuel up with sustainable carbs. Here's where you get your oomph. Your body breaks down carbohydrates in foods to give you stamina and mojo. But not all carbohydrates are created equal. There are two types—simple and complex. Simple carbs, also called simple sugars, are rapidly absorbed into your bloodstream, thereby leading to a fast jolt followed by plummeting energy levels. Think of candy or the white granulated sugar your mom used to keep in a jar on the kitchen counter. That said, you'll also find simple sugars in nutritious foods such as fruit and milk, and this is why those products are limited in KO-90. You won't be eating fruit for the first three months, but once you've lost 70 percent of your goal, you'll be able to start adding some back in; especially blueberries, which are high in antioxidants.

On the other side of the pantry, complex carbohydrates are ideal for keeping energy levels pumping. Choices like oatmeal; sweet potatoes; brown, black, or long-grain white rice; and whole-wheat couscous take longer to break down and be absorbed, so your blood-sugar levels don't spike and you're left with smooth, long-lasting fuel. These natural power sources are also rich in fiber, which keeps your digestive system humming and promotes a sense of fullness. That's why a medium-sized yam will fill you up better and longer than a peanut butter cup, even though both contain a similar number of calories.

Breads and pastas are also considered complex carbs, but they're often highly refined, meaning their nutrients and fiber have been stripped and removed, so steer away. Besides, controlling yourself around them can be too challenging; I've seen many a good day obliterated by a warm bread basket, and pasta is nearly always drenched in butter, oil, cream, or cheese.

I like to base carbohydrate intake around my clients' workouts. Keep the bulk of them in the first half of your day: oatmeal at breakfast and three Wasa flatbread crisps topped with canned tuna, tomato, and cucumber slices and cracked pepper for a mid-morning snack. Try to avoid carbs later in the day, when they are more likely to be stored as fat.

"Good" Carbs versus "Bad" Carbs

Certain foods cause your blood sugar to spike, delivering a fleeting hit of energy that is followed by a crash (e.g., naptime). Others infuse you with a steady stream of fuel. Guess which kind you want? Known as "Low Glycemic Index" foods, these items are high in fiber and slowly digested, so they won't take you on a blood-sugar roller coaster. KO-90 is low in carbs overall, but the carbs you *do* enjoy are low GI.

Is That a Cucumber in Your Pocket or Are You Just Happy to See Me?

Need yet another reason to up your veggie intake? People who eat healthy foods like peppers, carrots, and dark leafy greens are considered more attractive by their peers—sexier than someone with a tan even! When shown images of fifty-one faces and offered two ways to render the faces more attractive, subjects preferred the glow typically derived from eating carotenoids, a type of antioxidants found in produce, more than a traditional tan. The magic number: five servings a day will keep nights home alone away.[4]

LOW GLYCEMIC FOODS (HIGHLY RECOMMENDED)

Oatmeal

Low-starch vegetables (those listed in my Rock Star Produce list, page 52)

Long-grain white rice

Whole-wheat cereal

Beans

Nuts (in moderation)

HIGH GLYCEMIC FOODS (STEER CLEAR)

Potatoes

Bagels

Candy

Pasta

PJ's **Conquering Cravings**
Pointer

When I was trying to lose the weight and a craving struck, I knew I had to look within myself and recognize the fact that, even though the food might taste good in the moment, it wasn't worth the sluggishness and guilt I would feel afterward. I would literally tell myself, "PJ, sugar makes you feel like garbage ten minutes after you swallow it." Sometimes my craving would still win out, and then I'd have to encourage myself to accept the fact that I'd made a mistake and figure out a game plan for not getting myself into that same situation again. But I knew that even if I changed my eating habits by just one good decision per day, I'd eventually overpower the weight. Take responsibility for yourself: if you don't eat garbage, you'll feel better. When you feel better, you'll see results. And when you see results, you'll be motivated to keep making smart choices.

"When I heard my breakfast would be oats and water, the first thing I said was 'You've got to be kidding me.' But I swear—I cannot live without it now! Also, I come from a Greek background, and we love our olive oil and feta. Mediterranean cuisine can be very healthy but also unhealthy at the same time. But you learn to adjust, and once you start seeing the results, you become addicted to clean eating. I'm in the Maintenance Phase now, so I'm allowed to throw in a 'cheat' meal every so often, but you know what? I'd choose my lean steak with veggies over fast food any day! If you had told me a year ago that I would be saying this, I would never have believed it!"

—**Zoi Georgiou,** age twenty-five, lost 55 pounds

Power up with protein. In Australia kangaroo is a popular option. Not feeling that adventurous? Turn to seafood, chicken, turkey, lean red meat, and tofu for this crucial macro-

"I only found the clean eating plan difficult in the first week. After that it was more or less easy sailing. My cravings melted away within weeks of not feeding them."

—**Dr. John Parkes,** age sixty, lost 88 pounds

nutrient. Protein is a key component of every single cell in your body, from your hair and nails to your quads and lats to the blood coursing through your veins. It keeps your immune system humming and allows you to build and repair tissue. It's also incredibly satisfying, keeping you fuller, longer—thus spurring fat loss.

When choosing your proteins, you want to choose lean varieties to protect yourself from artery-clogging cholesterol and saturated fat. Avoid marbled cuts of beef and instead choose round, chuck, sirloin, or tenderloin. When purchasing ground beef, stay away from prepackaged varieties: even a package labeled "90 percent lean" can still pack a significant amount of fat. Instead, visit your local butcher and pick out a cut of meat you like, ask him to grind it in front of you, and maybe even have him shape it into four 5-ounce patties. Voila! Healthy hamburgers to grill whenever you like.

Ground chicken or turkey can contain as much or even more fat as ground beef because it often includes dark meat and skin, so repeat the process with your butcher or look for "extra lean" on the label. White-meat chicken or turkey is far leaner than dark meat, and you should always remove the skin, which is almost pure fat. As for fish, fatty selections like salmon are rich in heart-healthy omega 3 fatty acids, but your current goal is fat loss, so for the time being choose low-fat varieties of white fish, such as tilapia, cod, and flounder, saving the salmon for special celebrations in the maintenance phase of KO-90.

Drink up. Water does far more than simply quench your thirst; it comprises 60 percent of your body weight—keeping your energy levels up, carrying nutrients to cells, and flushing toxins out of organs. Unfortunately, many of us walk around in a chronic state of dehydration: either we forget to drink or we reach for other options because we find the taste of plain water to be boring.

A widespread recommendation is the "8 x 8" approach: drink eight 8-ounce glasses of water a day. If that motto works for you, great. But if it seems daunting, try instead to focus on drinking enough water that you never feel thirsty and your urine is pale yellow or clear. (Urine that looks like lemonade or beer is a sure sign of dehydration.) Even just 1 percent dehydration is enough to impair your performance in the gym, so really make an effort to stay on top of it. Remember, it doesn't have to be plain tap water: decaffeinated tea and coffee count, as does water flavored with lemon, lime, orange, or cucumber.

PJ's Pointer

Fill 'er Up

Drink one to two glasses of water before every meal. I found this helped me feel full without seeming overwhelming, as the standard "eight glasses a day" rule can feel.

Food counts too. According to the Institute of Medicine, 20 percent of our total water intake actually comes from juicy foods like vegetables, beans, oatmeal, chicken, and fish.[5] What's more, "eating" your water may be even smarter than drinking it because you reap the benefits of, say, the antioxidants in your celery or the protein in your fish.

Just say no. If you're serious about effective fat loss, you can't drink alcohol. Although a daily glass of wine has cardio-protective benefits, the empty calories and relaxing effect can promote overeating and negative food choices. Even worse, the food you consume while drinking beer, wine, or liquor is destined to be stored as fat because as your body works to metabolize alcohol, it diverts its attention and energy *away* from metabolizing your meal. Your thighs grow bigger as your blood-alcohol level returns to normal. Booze also lowers your blood sugar, thereby spurring hunger—and I defy you to tell me one time when you've been buzzed and decided to raid your fridge for carrot sticks.

Ditch the dairy. Many believe that dairy products are the best ways to get bone-strengthening calcium and immune system–enhancing Vitamin D; unfortunately, they're also excellent at causing bloat, thus contributing to what looks like a layer of liquid beneath the skin. By eliminating dairy from your diet, you'll see results more quickly and may find digestive and skin issues clear up as well. And here's the best part: you don't need to worry about calcium deficiencies because you can still derive plenty of calcium from broccoli and other leafy green vegetables, tofu, edamame, plus a daily calcium supplement. However, make sure you take it with a vitamin D supplement as well, which is difficult to obtain from food.

THE MEAL PLAN

My philosophy on eating is "Eat like the person you wish to become, not the person you are now."

For the first three months my clients follow a strict menu that stays fairly consistent from day to day. I have found that this is the best way to get people accustomed to a routine. Every day the meals will differ slightly—enough to offer a sense of variety without derailing your options with too many choices, mile-long grocery lists, or time-consuming preparation. People who are overweight tend to have poor time-management skills and when given too much flexibility, the results are nowhere near what they could be. Taking the thought process out of the equation helps deliver optimal results.

A WAIST OF BEVERAGE

Think diet soda will help you lose weight? Think again. In one new study, diet soft-drink users experience 70 percent greater increases in waist circumference compared with nondrinkers. Those who downed two or more diet sodas a day suffered from *500 percent* greater increases! Artificial sweeteners are super sweet, fooling your body into expecting an influx of calories. But when those calories don't arrive (because diet soda is calorie-free), you may become hungrier and wind up eating more.[6] Studies done on the increasing waistline measurements and spiraling glucose levels in mice have hinted toward sweeteners' effect—and the same goes for people.[7]

I want you to trust me here. A lot of these dishes are probably unlike what you're eating now. But stick with me and remember to take it one meal at a time. Pretty soon you'll begin stringing together multiple healthy meals and snacks, and you'll find yourself taking it one day at a time. Then one week at a time. Soon, the first ninety days will be over, and you'll have made it past the first—and most crucial—hurdle. At that point, if you're at or near your weight-loss goal, it will be time to transition to the Maintenance Phase, which will give you the opportunity to start re-introducing old favorites (preferably the *healthy* ones, such as fruit and nuts, but a burger here and there is perfectly acceptable). But I'm telling you—you *will* start to love eating clean and the way it makes you feel.

Many books will map out a month's worth of breakfasts, lunches, dinners, and snacks for you. But I want to teach you to stand on your own two feet. After reading *Take It Off, Keep It Off*, you'll feel strong enough and knowledgeable enough to pick and choose from the options I present to you. That way *you're* controlling *your* destiny; *I'm* not controlling *you*.

Here are a couple of notes about the recipes:

Power to the Protein.   You'll see some of the meals call for protein powder. This should be high-protein, low-carb, sugar-free, no-fat, and low-sodium powder; my clients use my Platinum Protein powder, available from www.pjapproved.com. When mixing protein powder into your oatmeal, be sure to add the boiling water first, followed by the protein powder when your oats cool down slightly.

It's All in the Seasoning.   In all of my recipes seasoning should be to taste—herbs are calorie- and sodium-free, so feel free to shake on a generous sprinkling, according to taste.

Morning Joe.   All coffee should contain no milk/cream or sugar/artificial sweetener.

Special Populations

Because men and women are built differently, I have provided two separate menus; the foods are the same, but the amounts are slightly different. Men will need 20 percent more fuel to accommodate for their added muscle mass—that is, if the women's menu plan specifies five ounces of fish, men will prepare and eat up to six ounces. Men, if your weight loss stalls and you are training and exercising correctly, this would suggest that the increase in food consumption is not ideal for you and you should instead follow the lower-calorie (women's) plan.

If you are morbidly obese (one hundred pounds or more above your ideal body weight), you will require more calories throughout the day. Be sure to consult a physician first to make sure you are healthy enough to begin the KO-90 plan. As for food, you can increase the amount of food in each of the three existing meals by 20 percent. So instead of eating 1.5 ounces of oats at breakfast, try 1.8; instead of topping three Wasa Crisps with 4 ounces of lean turkey and sliced cucumber and tomato for a midmorning snack, top them with 5 ounces of turkey. The important thing is that you don't become ravenous and risk being tempted by cravings. (If you find that increasing the amount of food stalls your weight loss, you've added too much.)

Women

DAY ONE

Breakfast

Sprinkle three large shredded-wheat biscuits with 1.5 ounces protein powder mixed with 7 ounces water. Serve with one cup of black coffee, green or herbal tea, or hot water with lemon.

Calories: 327

Morning Snack

Three Wasa Crisps topped with 4 ounces turkey breast and four slices of cucumber and tomato.

Calories: 242

Lunch

One small pita pocket filled with 3.5 ounces lean, grilled fillet steak, four tomato slices, grated carrot (1 ounce), and grilled red bell peppers (1 ounce).

Calories: 293

Afternoon Snack

One 3.5-ounce grilled chicken breast, served with 3 ounces oven-baked sweet potato and 3 ounces steamed broccoli.

Calories: 246

Late-Afternoon Snack

Mix 1.5 ounces protein powder with 8 ounces water.

Calories: 166

Dinner

One 5-ounce white-flesh fish fillet (tilapia, flounder, sea bass), seasoned with fresh rosemary and sprinkled with lemon juice, tightly wrapped in aluminum foil and baked on a tray with a shallow water bath (pour a small amount of water onto the tray, just enough to provide a thin barrier between the fish and the tray) at 350°F for twelve minutes. Serve with 3.5 ounces steamed spinach.

Calories: 157

DAY ONE TOTAL CALORIES: 1,431

DAY TWO

Breakfast

Mix 1.5 ounces oats with 7 ounces boiling water and 1.5 ounces protein powder. Serve with one cup of black coffee, green or herbal tea, or hot water with lemon.

Calories: 355

Morning Snack

Three Wasa Crisps topped with 4 ounces lean turkey breast and four slices of cucumber and tomato.

Calories: 242

Lunch

One small pita pocket filled with 4.5 ounces ratatouille mix (1 ounce each of diced eggplant, tomatoes, onions, zucchini, and bell peppers, with garlic, cracked pepper, and rosemary; place mix in a nonstick oven dish, cover with lid or aluminum foil, and bake at 300°F for sixty minutes or until cooked through; remove foil and allow to crisp in the oven for another ten minutes).

Calories: 150

Afternoon Snack

One 3.5-ounce grilled chicken breast, served with 3 ounces oven-baked sweet potato.

Calories: 221

Late-Afternoon Snack

Mix 1.5 ounces protein powder with 8 ounces water.

Calories: 166

Dinner

Two 2.5-ounce grilled fillet steak patties (ask your butcher to remove excess fat and shape ground meat into hamburger patties for grilling), seasoned with thyme. Wrap each patty in lettuce and top with 3.5 ounces sliced mushrooms, sautéed with crushed garlic.

Calories: 318

DAY TWO TOTAL CALORIES: 1,454

You'll notice that your evening meals typically don't include heavy carbs. Oatmeal, rice, shredded wheat, crackers, pita bread, and sweet potatoes are all encouraged—but primarily early in the day. I would never recommend a zero-carb diet, which would result in your body going into starvation mode, holding on to everything you eat and preventing the body from effectively burning calories. But in moderation, carbs keep your energy up and your metabolism humming, and by consuming most carbs before 2 p.m. you give your body its best chance at burning them off. Basically, you'll teach your body to use less energy throughout the day because it senses the upcoming reduction in calories and compensates by working more efficiently.

DAY THREE

Breakfast

Three large shredded-wheat biscuits sprinkled with 1.5 ounces protein powder mixed with 7 ounces water. Serve with one cup of black coffee, green or herbal tea, or hot water with lemon.

Calories: 327

Morning Snack

Chicken salad: mix 4 ounces grilled, cubed chicken with 1 ounce each cucumber, red peppers, Spanish onion, and tomato, plus 1 tablespoon Dijon mustard and cilantro to taste.

Calories: 244

Lunch

Three Wasa Crisps spread with 3 ounces mashed sweet potato and topped with 4 ounces thinly sliced grilled lean beef.

Calories: 372

Afternoon Snack

Two hard-boiled eggs, cut in half and seasoned with cracked pepper. Serve with small handful of celery and carrot sticks (five of each, four inches long).

Calories: 167

Late-Afternoon Snack

Mix 1.5 ounces protein powder with 8 ounces water.

Calories: 166

Dinner

One 5-ounce white-flesh fish (tilapia, flounder, sea bass), seasoned with tarragon and two to three thin slices of lime and sprinkled with a dash of water, wrapped in aluminum foil and baked on a tray with a shallow water bath at 350°F for fourteen minutes or until cooked through. Serve with 3.5 ounces steamed broccoli.

Calories: 157

DAY THREE TOTAL CALORIES: 1,433

PJ's Pointer

I know what you're thinking: I-M-P-O-S-S-I-B-L-E. Starvation diet. Worse than rabbit food. Who does this guy think he is? But hear me out: yes, it's challenging. Yes, it may be the toughest thing you'll ever do. But trust me—it *will* work. It's actually not uncommon for my clients to tell me that the sheer volume of food feels a bit overwhelming—the opposite of feeling deprived. That's because many overweight people are accustomed to consuming calorie-dense foods, like deep-dish pizza and cheeseburgers. But here, the foods are low calorie but high volume, so despite all of the salads and vegetables, you absolutely will feel full and satisfied. All of my clients stick to this eating plan, or something very similar, even after they have reached their goal weight because they love the ease of it and the positive effect it has on their mood and energy levels.

DAY FOUR

Breakfast

Three large shredded-wheat biscuits sprinkled with 1.5 ounces protein powder mixed with 7 ounces water. Serve with one cup of black coffee, green or herbal tea, or hot water with lemon.

Calories: 327

Morning Snack

Three Wasa Crisps topped with 4 ounces lean turkey breast and four slices of cucumber and tomato.

Calories: 242

Lunch

Season 4 ounces grilled chicken with paprika powder and make into a salad with 1 ounce each of cucumber, red peppers, Spanish onion, and tomato, and 1 teaspoon Dijon mustard (no extra oil).

Calories: 244

Afternoon Snack

Veggie stir-fry (1 ounce each of broccoli, mushrooms, red onion, carrot, and tofu, all cut into bite-sized chunks, and bean shoots), sautéed with a small amount of spray olive oil and tossed with 1 level tablespoon crushed, unsalted peanuts. Serve on a bed of 3 ounces long-grain white rice.

Calories: 228

Late-Afternoon Snack

Mix 1.5 ounces protein powder with 8 ounces water.

Calories: 166

Dinner

One 5-ounce tuna steak fillet, sautéed in a small amount of olive oil spray and topped with 1 to 2 teaspoons of ground, fresh red chili paste to taste and drizzled with lemon juice. Serve with 3 ounces steamed string beans.

Calories: 260

DAY FOUR TOTAL CALORIES: 1,467

Did you notice that you get three snacks per day? Something tells me that might be more than you eat now—am I right? These midmorning and afternoon nibbles are more like mini-meals, stoking your furnace (i.e., your stomach) and keeping your metabolism humming along. They're all mainly protein based, which means they're incredibly satisfying while contributing relatively few calories. Some of my clients' favorites include hard-boiled eggs seasoned with cracked pepper (not just one—you get two!); freshly made chicken salad; Wasa Crisps topped with lean turkey breast, cucumber, and tomato; and veggie stir-fry served over rice.

DAY FIVE

Breakfast

Mix 1.5 ounces oatmeal with 7 ounces boiling water and 1.5 ounces protein powder. Serve with one cup of black coffee, green or herbal tea, or hot water with lemon.

Calories: 355

Morning Snack

Tuna salad: 4 ounces spring water–packed tuna mixed with 1 ounce each tomato, cucumber, and celery, as much lettuce as you like, and 1 teaspoon balsamic vinegar.

Calories: 187

Lunch

One 3.5-ounce chicken breast, seasoned with turmeric and cooked on the grill or baked in a pan sprayed with a small amount of olive oil spray, served with 3 ounces long-grain white rice and 3 ounces steamed asparagus spears tossed with one clove of crushed garlic.

Calories: 283

Afternoon Snack

One 4-ounce grilled fillet steak, seasoned with oregano and chili powder, served with one small ripe tomato cut in wedges and one sliced cucumber.

Calories: 244

Late-Afternoon Snack

Mix 1.5 ounces protein powder with 8 ounces water.

Calories: 166

Dinner

One 3.5-ounce chicken breast seasoned with Cajun spices, cooked on the grill or baked in a pan with a small amount of olive oil spray. Serve with 3 ounces oven-baked sweet potato and 3 ounces steamed broccoli.

Calories: 246

DAY FIVE TOTAL CALORIES: 1,481

DAY SIX

Breakfast

Three large shredded-wheat biscuits sprinkled with 1.5 ounces protein powder and 7 ounces water. Serve with one cup of black coffee, green or herbal tea, or hot water with lemon.

Calories: 327

Morning Snack

One 4-ounce grilled chicken breast, served with 3 ounces cooked long-grain white rice and 3 ounces steamed broccoli.

Calories: 317

Lunch

Tuna salad: 4 ounces spring water–packed tuna, 1 ounce each tomato, cucumber, and celery, as much lettuce as you like, and 1 tablespoon balsamic vinegar.

Calories: 187

Afternoon Snack

Two hard-boiled eggs, cut in half and seasoned with cracked pepper. Serve with small handful of celery and carrot sticks (five of each, four inches long).

Calories: 167

Late-Afternoon Snack

Mix 1.5 ounces protein powder with 8 ounces water.

Calories: 166

Dinner

One 5-ounce white-flesh fish fillet (tilapia, flounder, sea bass), seasoned with tarragon, sprinkled with lemon juice, wrapped in aluminum foil, and baked on a tray with a shallow water bath at 350°F for fourteen minutes or until cooked through.

Serve with 3 ounces sweet potato fries (cut sweet potato into French fry shape or wedges; add whole cloves of garlic and rosemary sprigs and then season with cracked pepper, cumin, and half teaspoon of extra-virgin olive oil; bake on nonstick tray at 400°F for thirty minutes or until crispy and cooked through) and 3 ounces steamed, mixed vegetables (try a trio of red, yellow, and green bell peppers).

Calories: 251

DAY SIX TOTAL CALORIES: 1,415

DAY SEVEN

Breakfast

Mix 1.5 ounces oatmeal with 7 ounces boiling water and 1.5 ounces protein powder. Serve with one cup of black coffee, green or herbal tea, or hot water with lemon.

Calories: 355

Morning Snack

Three Wasa Crisps topped with 4 ounces lean turkey breast and four slices of cucumber and tomato.

Calories: 242

Lunch

Tuna salad: 4 ounces spring water–packed tuna, 1 ounce each tomato, cucumber, and celery, as much lettuce as you like, and 1 tablespoon balsamic vinegar.

Calories: 187

PJ's Pointer — The Most Important Meal of the Day

I see it all the time: clients think that by skipping breakfast they're starting the day off "right"—with a calorie deficit. I fell into that mental trap too when I was trying to lose weight—partly because rolling out of bed and heading right to work was easier and partly because, despite my education and knowledge, I convinced myself that doing so would save me calories. But by 10 a.m. my stomach would be growling like a bear, and no amount of salad or tuna fish could satisfy it. After about a month I wised up and started eating a healthy breakfast. My morning hunger pangs quieted, I had *way* more energy and was able to make smarter decisions at lunch and dinner. Don't ditch breakfast: your metabolism will thank you.

Afternoon Snack

One 3.5-ounce grilled chicken breast, marinated in crushed garlic and turmeric to taste, served with 3 ounces oven-baked sweet potato.

Calories: 221

Late-Afternoon Snack

Mix 1.5 ounces protein powder with 8 ounces water.

Calories: 166

Dinner

One 5-ounce rib-eye steak (remove any fat), seasoned with oregano and cracked black pepper and grilled or baked in a pan with a small amount of olive oil spray. Serve with 3.5 ounces steamed mixed vegetables (bok choy or mushrooms and onions would be a tasty complement to the steak).

Calories: 300

DAY SEVEN TOTAL CALORIES: 1,471

Men

DAY ONE

Breakfast

Sprinkle 3.5 large shredded-wheat biscuits with 1.8 ounces protein powder mixed with 7 ounces water. Serve with one cup of black coffee, green or herbal tea, or hot water with lemon.

Calories: 392

Morning Snack

Top 3.5 Wasa Crisps with 5 ounces lean turkey breast and five slices of cucumber and tomato.

Calories: 290

Lunch

One small pita pocket filled with 4.5 ounces lean, grilled fillet steak, five tomato slices, grated carrot (1.5 ounces), and grilled red bell peppers (1.5 ounces).

Calories: 352

Afternoon Snack

One 4.5-ounce grilled chicken breast, served with 3.5 ounces oven-baked sweet potato and 3.5 ounces steamed broccoli.

Calories: 295

Late-Afternoon Snack

Mix 1.8 ounces protein powder with 8 ounces water.

Calories: 199

Dinner

One 6-ounce white-flesh fish (tilapia, flounder, sea bass), seasoned with fresh rosemary and sprinkled with lemon juice, wrapped in aluminum foil and baked on a tray with a shallow water bath at 350°F for fourteen minutes. Serve with 4.5 ounces steamed spinach.

Calories: 188

DAY ONE TOTAL CALORIES: 1,716

DAY TWO

Breakfast

Mix 2 ounces oatmeal with 7 ounces boiling water and 1.8 ounces protein powder. Serve with one cup of black coffee, green or herbal tea, or hot water with lemon.

Calories: 426

Morning Snack

Top 3.5 Wasa Crisps with 5 ounces lean turkey breast and five slices of cucumber and tomato.

Calories: 290

Lunch

One small pita pocket filled with 5.5 ounces ratatouille mix (1.5 ounce each diced eggplant, tomatoes, onions, zucchini, and bell peppers, with garlic, cracked pepper, and rosemary; place mix in a nonstick oven dish, cover with lid or aluminum foil, and bake at 300°F for sixty minutes or until cooked through; remove foil and allow to crisp in the oven for another ten minutes).

Calories: 180

Afternoon Snack

One 4.5-ounce grilled chicken breast, served with 3.5 ounces oven-baked sweet potato.

Calories: 265

Late-Afternoon Snack

Mix 1.8 ounces protein powder with 8 ounces water.

Calories: 199

Dinner

Two 3-ounce grilled fillet steak patties (ask your butcher to remove excess fat and shape ground meat into hamburger patties for grilling), seasoned with fresh thyme. Wrap each patty in lettuce together with 4.5 ounces sliced mushrooms, sautéed with crushed garlic.

Calories: 382

DAY TWO TOTAL CALORIES: 1,742

DAY THREE

Breakfast

Sprinkle 3.5 large shredded-wheat biscuits sprinkled with 1.8 ounces protein powder and 7 ounces water. Serve with one cup of black coffee, green or herbal tea, or hot water with lemon.

Calories: 392

Morning Snack

Chicken salad: mix 4.8 ounces grilled, cubed chicken with 1.5 ounce each cucumber, red peppers, Spanish onion, and tomato, plus 1 teaspoon Dijon mustard and cilantro to taste.

Calories: 293

Lunch

Spread 3.5 Wasa Crisps with 3.5 ounces mashed sweet potato and top with 5 ounces thinly sliced grilled lean beef.

Calories: 446

Afternoon Snack

Cut 2.5 hard-boiled eggs in half and season with cracked pepper. Serve with one handful of celery and carrot sticks (six of each, four inches long).

Calories: 200

Late-Afternoon Snack

Mix 1.8 ounces protein powder with 8 ounces water.

Calories: 199

Dinner

One 6-ounce white-flesh fish fillet (tilapia, flounder, sea bass), seasoned with fresh tarragon and thinly sliced lime and sprinkled with a dash of water, wrapped in aluminum foil, and baked on a tray with a shallow water bath at 350°F for fourteen minutes or until cooked through. Serve with 4.5 ounces steamed broccoli.

Calories: 188

DAY THREE TOTAL CALORIES: 1,718

DAY FOUR

Breakfast

Sprinkle 3.5 large shredded-wheat biscuits with 1.8 ounces protein powder and 7 ounces water. Serve with one cup of black coffee, green or herbal tea, or hot water with lemon.

Calories: 392

Morning Snack

Top 3.5 Wasa Crisps with 5 ounces lean turkey breast and five slices of cucumber and tomato.

Calories: 290

PJ's Pointer Get Cooking

To save time I cook a big batch of rice at the beginning of the week and then divide it into individual preportioned containers and store them in the refrigerator. That way, when a recipe calls for rice, I don't need to spend time heating up and boiling the water, cooking and straining the rice—I can just grab and prepare. Another tip: cook your rice just about three-quarters of the way done. It will keep cooking a little bit in the fridge as it cools down, and mushy rice doesn't exactly scream "Delicious!" Apply this to sweet potato as well.

Lunch

Season 5 ounces grilled chicken with paprika powder and make into a salad with 1.5 ounces each cucumber, red peppers, Spanish onion, and tomato, and 1 teaspoon Dijon mustard (no oil).

Calories: 293

Afternoon Snack

Veggie stir-fry (1.5 ounces each of broccoli, mushrooms, red onion, carrot, and tofu, all cut into bite-sized chunks, and bean shoots), sautéed with a small amount of spray olive oil and tossed with 1 level teaspoon crushed, unsalted peanuts. Serve on a bed of 3.5 ounces long-grain white rice.

Calories: 274

Late-Afternoon Snack

Mix 1.8 ounces protein powder with 8 ounces water.

Calories: 199

Dinner

One 6-ounce tuna steak fillet, sautéed in a small amount of olive oil spray and topped with ground, fresh red chili paste to taste and drizzled with lemon juice. Serve with 3.5 ounces steamed string beans.

Calories: 312

DAY FOUR TOTAL CALORIES: 1,760

DAY FIVE

Breakfast

Mix 2 ounces oatmeal with 7 ounces boiling water and 1.8 ounces protein powder. Serve with one cup of black coffee, green or herbal tea, or hot water with lemon.

Calories: 426

Morning Snack

Tuna salad: 5 ounces spring water–packed tuna mixed with 1.5 ounces each tomato, cucumber, and celery, as much lettuce as you like, and 1 teaspoon balsamic vinegar.

Calories: 224

Lunch

One 4.5-ounce chicken breast, seasoned with turmeric and cooked on the grill or baked in a pan sprayed with a small amount of olive oil spray. Serve with 3.5 ounces long-grain white rice and 3.5 ounces steamed asparagus spears, tossed with one clove crushed garlic.

Calories: 340

Afternoon Snack

One 5-ounce grilled fillet steak, seasoned with oregano and chili powder and served with one small ripe tomato, cut in wedges, and one sliced cucumber.

Calories: 290

Late-Afternoon Snack

Mix 1.8 ounces protein powder with 8 ounces water.

Calories: 199

Dinner

One 4.5-ounce grilled chicken breast seasoned with Cajun spices and served with 3.5 ounces oven-baked sweet potato and 3.5 ounces steamed broccoli.

Calories: 295

DAY FIVE TOTAL CALORIES: 1,774

DAY SIX

Breakfast

Sprinkle 3.5 large shredded-wheat biscuits with 1.8 ounces protein powder and 7 ounces water. Serve with one cup of black coffee, green or herbal tea, or hot water with lemon.

Calories: 392

Morning Snack

One 5-ounce grilled chicken breast over 3.5 ounces cooked long-grain white rice, served with 3.5 ounces steamed broccoli.

Calories: 380

Lunch

Tuna salad: 5 ounces spring water–packed tuna, 1.5 ounces each tomato, cucumber, and celery, as much lettuce as you like, and 1 teaspoon balsamic vinegar.

Calories: 224

Afternoon Snack

2.5 hard-boiled eggs seasoned with cracked pepper. Serve with small handful of celery and carrot sticks (six of each, four inches long).

Calories: 200

Late-Afternoon Snack

Mix 1.8 ounces protein powder with 8 ounces water.

Calories: 199

Dinner

One 6-ounce white-flesh fish fillet (tilapia, flounder, sea bass), seasoned with herbs, sprinkled with lemon juice, wrapped in aluminum foil, and baked on a tray with a shallow water bath at 350°F for fourteen minutes or until cooked through. Serve with 3.5 ounces sweet potato fries (cut sweet potato into French fry shape or wedges; add whole cloves of garlic and rosemary sprigs and season with cracked pepper, cumin, and half teaspoon of extra-virgin olive oil; bake on nonstick tray at 400°F for thirty-five minutes or until crispy and cooked through) and 3.5 ounces steamed, mixed vegetables.

Calories: 301

DAY SIX TOTAL CALORIES: 1,696

DAY SEVEN

Breakfast

Mix 2 ounces oatmeal with 7 ounces boiling water and 1.8 ounces protein powder. Serve with one cup of black coffee, green or herbal tea, or hot water with lemon.

Calories: 426

Morning Snack

Top 3.5 Wasa Crisps with 5 ounces lean turkey breast and five slices of cucumber and tomato.

Calories: 290

Lunch

Tuna salad: 4.8 ounces spring water–packed tuna, 1.5 ounces each tomato, cucumber, and celery, as much lettuce as you like, and 1 teaspoon balsamic vinegar.

Calories: 224

Afternoon Snack

One 5-ounce grilled chicken breast, marinated in crushed garlic and turmeric, and served with 3.5 ounces oven-baked sweet potato.

Calories: 265

Late-Afternoon Snack

Mix 1.8 ounces protein powder with 8 ounces water.

Calories: 199

Dinner

One 6-ounce grilled rib-eye steak (remove any fat), seasoned with oregano, and served with 4.5 ounces steamed mixed vegetables.

Calories: 360

DAY SEVEN TOTAL CALORIES: 1,764

PJ's
Pointer

Rather than look at these menus and think, "There's so much to follow," instead, tell yourself, "All the work has already been done for me." I've taken the thinking out of eating for you—just eat what I've outlined here and don't worry about coming up with creative recipes or studying up on healthy preparation methods. Once you've gotten the hang of the program, you'll start understanding *why* these meals work (because you'll be losing weight while feeling satisfied), and I'll bet you start *wanting* to research and share inventive new recipes!

PREP SCHOOL

Between work, family, kids, friends, volunteering, and your new ramped-up workout routine, finding time to prepare your meals can be challenging. As a result, the drive-thru might start calling your name or you'll find yourself tempted to head straight for the refrigerator after a long day and eat anything you can get your hands on. Because of this, you need to prepare your kitchen so it works to your advantage in these types of situations. I found that if I had the bones of my meals prepared (individually portioned meat and chicken in the freezer; washed and cut-up produce in the fridge), lunch and dinner were infinitely easier to prepare, reducing the temptation to order Chinese take-out. I also had to force myself to rid my cupboards of cookies, chips, candy, and other junk food; the effort it took to resist those foods, knowing they were within arm's reach, was simply too great. Preparation is the key to staying out of trouble and will pave your way to success.

THE TARGET THEORY

Have you ever walked into a Target store with plans to purchase one or two items . . . and actually left with only one or two items? It's impossible! No one emerges from that store with just a bottle of shampoo or just a box of fabric softener. How about the food court at the mall? After hours of shopping, why does it always seem so tough to navigate away from Wendy's and Cinnabon? It's because having to make too many decisions weakens your willpower.[8] It's why even someone with the healthiest intentions can go into Baskin Robbins, hell-bent on ordering just a small scoop of raspberry sorbet, then get derailed by the other thirty-one flavors. Another example: between appetizers, drinks, meals, and desserts, the Cheesecake Factory's menu contains more than two hundred items, from the Cajun Jambalaya Pasta to the Barbeque Ranch Chicken Salad. You might think poring over such a limitless list would offer you a better chance of finding—and sticking with—a healthier entrée. But all that variety renders it difficult to stay focused on your goal.

That's why I'm a big fan of the KISS principle: Keep It Simple, Stupid. You need to rein in your meal and snack options to a core group of healthy foods—primarily those discussed above in "Rock Star Produce" and "Low Glycemic Foods." Sticking to a more select menu will help you reach your goals in a number of ways. First, it keeps the crap out of your house. My clients always—not often, but *always*—find that if they don't bring ice cream, chips, cookies, or candy into their homes, they are highly unlikely to venture out to purchase it, knowing it will only derail their efforts. Second, treating your fridge and pantry like an exclusive club (no losers allowed) frees up self-control and can actually help strengthen your resolve when it comes to tackling healthy activities later in the day, like hitting the gym or ignoring a coworker's candy dish.

You may think the word "regimented" has negative connotations, but when it comes to taking off weight, a reined-in grocery list is your best friend. Keeping your menu simple will free up self-control for other areas of your life, paving the way for a successful day.

PJ's Pointer

According to the US National Institutes of Health Division of Nutrition Research Coordination, the average person makes over 200 decisions about food every day.[9] That's 200-plus opportunities you have to make smart decisions. If you don't choose wisely for one, don't beat yourself up over it—you have 199 more chances to turn things around throughout the day.

STICKING TO THE PLAN

You may be tempted to follow these guidelines most—but not all—of the time or to pick and choose certain aspects that appeal to you ("I'll eliminate dairy but I need my fruit"). Be aware that by doing so you'll be cheating yourself out of your fullest potential. During my first two and a half months I actually lost very little weight—maybe ten pounds—because I was only following the plan 50 percent of the time. Guess what? When you commit to something 50 percent, you only get a 50 percent return—and that's if you're lucky. I thought losing the weight would be easy in light of my years of consistent exercising, but I had become heavily addicted to junk food and my body didn't want to let go of the weight. I thought I was special and would outperform my clients, but I wasn't—and I didn't.

Once I did buckle down and follow this plan to a T, however, the weight actually came off quite quickly. In that one month time period that followed I shed double the amount I'd lost in the prior two and a half months combined and the weight continued coming off all the way to the finish line. So when a client tells me, "I've been following the plan 75 percent of the time" and then they get on the scales to see they've lost about half of what they should have, only one of us is surprised.

I didn't have anyone pushing me and motivating me to succeed. But *you* have *me*. I want you to succeed, and I don't want the process to take any longer than it needs to. The plan might seem overwhelming at first, but I encourage you to accept the challenge. Think about all you have to gain by losing: more energy; increased self-esteem and confidence; a longer, healthier life; fewer sick days at work; less money spent on medical bills—the benefits go on and on. Isn't all that worth sacrificing your daily latte and Happy Hour cocktails?

Effective fat loss and body transformation requires a daily commitment from the time you begin until the time you reach your goal. There are no short cuts. If your goal is just losing weight rather than gaining overall health, this is the wrong book for you.

LOSING THE LAST 10 PERCENT

Once you've achieved 90 percent of your total weight-loss goal, it's time to start reintroducing some different types of foods—think good fats like nuts and avocado as well as fruit or whole-wheat pasta. This might sound counterintuitive—"How can adding in food help me lose more weight?"—but it is absolutely crucial. Your metabolism has a memory. Over time your body will become accustomed to processing clean food. Although that sounds good, it's actually slightly dangerous because your metabolism can grow lazy. And as you lose more and more weight, your body will enter panic mode and begin holding on to fat as a survival tactic. As a result people often find that their weight loss stalls with just 10 percent of their goal remaining. By feeding it something foreign, like a banana or some peanut butter or dressing with olive oil and vinegar, you're essentially tricking your metabolism into working overtime, thereby helping you lose more weight.

By the time you get to within 10 percent of your goal weight, your body will be an efficient, finely tuned machine. It's a great position to be in. The secret to incorporating a few "bad" or "missed" foods back into your eating plan? Do it only twice a week. For example, select one breakfast or lunch and one dinner (preferably three to four days apart). On these two occasions enjoy a meal of your choice that is not part of KO-90. It might be a PB&J, a big bowl of fruit, or scrambled eggs on toast with bacon. Stick to moderate portions—this is not a free pass to be gluttonous!—and really enjoy the foods; there's no reason to feel guilty. Eat the pasta or pizza and then immediately return to the menu plan for the next few days until it's time for the next scheduled treat. Your body will be confused by the sudden influx of calories and start burning more efficiently throughout the week. As long as you continue with your cardio and weights, you will push past the barrier and meet your goal.

Once you reach your goal weight—and you *will* reach your goal weight—you'll be able to add back even more "forbidden foods," such as a glass of merlot with dinner, a sandwich made with a whole-wheat wrap, or a low-fat yogurt topped with fruit. (Although, as I've said before, most of my clients are so enamored with their new bodies that they prefer to keep eating as cleanly as possible.) This will be considered your Maintenance Phase. It's much easier to maintain a body than to transform it. And you won't be prone to overindulging because after working so hard to get to this point, you'll be more inclined to watch yourself and protect your investment. If you do overdo it food-wise, you'll need to put in extra time at the gym, and you don't want that! I know I don't. ☺

Top 5 Faves — PJ's Pointer

Once you've neared your goal weight, make a Top 5 list of foods you'd love to reintroduce.

Eventually you will be able to enjoy that deep-dish again—but you'll possess the tools and knowledge needed to have a reasonable portion, satisfy your craving, and move on. I created my own list when I had just twelve pounds to go:

PJ's Top 5 List
Spaghetti carbonara
Pizza
Pork-filled dumplings
Gummi Bears
White chocolate

"Within three months I went from taking taxis to the gym to walking an 8K. I have more energy than ever before and look better at thirty-five than I did at twenty-five. I feel like I've been given a second chance in life. I try to forget that I wasted ten years eating and secluding myself from others. I feel so proud to have achieved something that, for many years, seemed impossible to control."
—Dora Dogas, age thirty-five, lost 198 pounds . . . and counting

At your goal weight you will be in full control—the master of your own destiny. You'll have given yourself a second chance at life. Don't waste it. You *can* be that man or woman on the beach who's in awesome shape, eating a cheeseburger—the one whose metabolism everyone else envies. What they don't know is how disciplined you are every other day of the week. Let others be envious of you, because, after all, they too have a choice. Be proud of yourself and what you have achieved. You too had a choice, and you chose life—so live it.

A NOTE ON VEGETARIAN DISHES

Although KO-90 is packed with fresh produce and even includes a few meat-free dishes, such as vegetable ratatouille, you'll notice that nearly every lunch and dinner includes some kind of animal protein, be it fish, chicken, or lean beef. That's by design: High amounts of protein are crucial to building muscle mass—one key factor in my approach to getting lean. The iron in meat also plays a role in helping your blood carry oxygen to tissues and keeping your energy surging. I've trained vegetarian clients in the past and have watched as they sabotaged themselves with meals that were high in carbs, fat, salt, sugar, and dairy and severely lacking in protein. To control for this they've had to resort to extra cardio, which runs counter to my policy of minimizing cardio to no more than fifteen minutes per session. These clients also struggled with fatigue due to low iron and vitamin B12 levels. I've even worked as a chef in vegetarian restaurants and have seen the amount of salt and fat that often gets poured into "healthy" meat-free options. That's not to say that truly healthy, thriving vegetarians don't exist—they do—but it takes a huge amount of planning, cooking and nutrition knowledge, and dedication. Having said that, I encourage those of you who are vegetarian to adopt the training strategies in this book. As for the food, tofu is an excellent source of protein for vegetarians, and many of the meat dishes can be substituted with tofu. When making choices, be mindful of hidden carbohydrates, fats, and sugars in seemingly "healthy" vegetarian foods. Being vegetarian simply means that you have to find clever ways to get the right ratio of protein to carbohydrates to fat in your eating plan. Difficult? Yes! Impossible? Never!

CHEATERS NEVER WIN

Plenty of diet and fitness plans offer a cheat day. It's usually a Saturday or Sunday (or both) when rules fly out the window and more indulgent foods are permitted. When I was first losing weight (or trying to, anyhow), I lived for my cheat day. Unfortunately, I had become totally addicted to fatty, salty foods and was completely lacking in discipline; in my eyes, every day was "Cheat Day"!

With an emphasis on eating clean and attaining optimum results, KO-90 does not include cheat days. I find that allowing clients cheat days from the outset gives a false sense of satisfaction; straying off course even once a week is enough to hinder your efforts. Your body and weight will plateau and you'll grow disillusioned, thinking the plan isn't working and causing you to throw your hands up in defeat. Eating clean 24–7 reinforces positive habits and commitment and ensures consistent results. That leads to a sense of authentic satisfaction and reward for all of your hard work. Follow my eating plan with the knowledge that you *will* be able to reintroduce some of your favorite foods once your metabolism has kicked in and your body can accommodate a few more calories without compromising fat loss.

But even then it won't be so much a "Cheat Day" as a "Cheat Meal." In fact, I've never had a client practice regular "Cheat Days" . . . and trust me, plenty of them *beg* for them—in the beginning. That's because their mindset has changed: after losing the weight, they're so happy with their progress that they never want to go back to how they used to feel when eating a full day's worth of "cheat" food—not even the most stubborn junk-food addict who

> **SUCCESS STORY SUZANNE**
>
> *"Apart from the practical stuff, like eating clean, focusing on my workouts, planning meals, and believing in myself, the best advice PJ has given me deals with eating out at restaurants. He tells me to enjoy it, not to feel guilty, and just to get back on track the next day."*
>
> —**Suzanne Konstantinides**, age forty-six, lost 33 pounds . . . and counting

claims he can't wait to hit his goal weight so he can reward himself with pasta, burgers, French fries, and beer. The further you come with your body, the further you'll want to distance yourself from your old one. Likewise, the better shape you achieve, the better your chances for indulging in a few "cheat" meals here and there without it affecting you in the long run.

When you do indulge, do so in a controlled fashion. If it's your birthday and you want to celebrate with a slice of cake, that's understandable . . . but don't binge on three slices and take home extra slices for breakfast tomorrow. Enjoy the treat and move on, knowing you'll need to spend some extra time in the gym later that day. Oh, and Happy Birthday!

A TYPICAL CLIENT MEAL—BEFORE AND AFTER

Most people aren't aware of just how many calories they are consuming on a daily basis. When I take on a new client, I always ask them to keep track of a day's worth of food and drink. Here's an example of what I'm often presented with.

Usually, the person professes to have been on a health kick over the past few weeks and he or she is very excited to show me their new and improved "healthy eating plan." They truly think they've instigated some positive changes and are eager to impress me with their eating plan—but almost always, their meals and snacks are still quite high in sneaky sources of fat, sugar, salt, and carbs. (When I ask them what they were eating before the recent health kick, that's when the pizza, burgers, fries, alcohol, chips, candy, and cake come out.) The following example shows how, in general, people lack a true understanding of what it means to eat healthy:

BEGINNING CLIENT'S "HEALTHY" CHOICE MENU
(before I meet with them)

Breakfast
Two ounces granola, with fruit and nut pieces, topped with 7 ounces low-fat milk, chocolate-chip granola bar, 4 ounces plain yogurt, and medium latte, no sugar.

Calories: 699

Morning Snack
One 4-ounce tuna salad with 8.5-ounce carton apple juice.

Calories: 408

Lunch
Subway 6-inch turkey sub (no dressing) with 20-ounce Coke Zero.

Calories: 256

Afternoon Snack
Small protein shake (low carb) mixed with 8.5 ounces low-fat milk.

Calories: 266

Dinner

Grilled 9-ounce T-bone steak, mashed potatoes, steamed vegetables, two glasses red wine.

Calories: 818

TOTAL CALORIES FOR THE DAY: 2,447

Now, compare that with a typical day on KO-90:

MY MENU

Breakfast

Two ounces raw oats with 7 ounces water and 1.5-ounce scoop protein powder, served with one cup black coffee.

Calories: 499

Morning Snack

Three Wasa Crisps topped with 3.5 ounces lean turkey breast and four medium slices cucumber and tomato.

Calorics: 217

Lunch

Tuna salad (3 ounces spring water–packed tuna with tomato, cucumber, lettuce, celery, and balsamic vinegar).

Calories: 95

Afternoon Snack

Onc 3.5-ounce grilled chicken breast with 3 ounces oven-baked sweet potato.

Calories: 221

Late-Afternoon Snack

Small protein shake with 8 ounces water.

Calories: 166

Dinner

Grilled 5-ounce rib-eye steak with steamed vegetables.

Calories: 300

TOTAL CALORIES FOR THE DAY: 1,498

In the "before" case a person would be consuming an extra:

- 949 calories over the course of one day,
- 6,643 calories over the course of one week, and
- 345,436 calories over the course of one year.

At 200 pounds, to burn off 6,643 weekly calories, you would need to:

- swim freestyle, continuously, for 10.5 hours,
- walk at a moderate pace for 22 hours,
- use the Elliptical trainer at a low pace for nearly 7.5 hours,
- ride a Spin bike—hard—for 13.5 hours, or
- lift weights with low intensity for 25 hours.

Even if you *did* somehow manage to burn off all those extra calories in the week, you'll simply end up where you were at the start of the week—out of shape and unmotivated to do anything about it (not to mention dead from exhaustion).

You can play around with figures all day long, but the one figure you really should be focusing on is your own.

PANTRY RAID!

In order to prepare healthy meals, you need to own a healthy kitchen. What's a healthy kitchen? It's stocked with equipment and gadgets that enable you to cook low-fat, low-cal meals and snacks that don't taste like cardboard.

One crucial tool: a food scale. Weighing your food will teach you proper portion control. The amount of food that restaurants heap on our plates has radically skewed our views on what is an appropriate amount of food. True, fine French dining establishments will present you with a small portion of meat, and authentic Italian cooking calls for relatively spare mounds of pasta. But midscale restaurants—the kind most of America eats at—serve monstrous portions that will only get you into trouble. When you start measuring your food, stick to:

Meat/fish/poultry. 3.5–5 ounces for women and 4.5–6 ounces for men (raw).

TAKE IT OFF,

Vegetables. 2–4 ounces for women and 4–6 ounces for men (raw).

Carbohydrates. 3 ounces raw sweet potato, 1.5 ounces dry oatmeal, 3 ounces cooked rice for women, and 3.5–4 ounces raw sweet potato, 2–3 ounces dry oatmeal, 3.5–4 ounces cooked rice for men.

After two or three weeks, you'll feel confident enough to put the scales away and will be able to accurately eyeball the proper amount of food.

The following are all tools I personally use in my own home kitchen. I urge you to visit your local kitchen and home goods store and stock up. Think of it as an investment in your health.

Healthy Kitchen Tools

Steamer. Allows you to cook vegetables and fish without any added fat.

Grill pan. Another clean way to prepare vegetables, meat, poultry, and fish; fat in the meat will drip down.

Immersion blender. Great for whipping up satisfying homemade vegetable soups, right in the pot.

Microplane. For grating tangy citrus zest over seafood and vegetables.

Garlic press. Delivers mouthwatering, calorie- and fat-free flavor without smelly hands.

Wok. For easy stir-fries; make sure it has a nonstick coating so you don't need much oil.

Oil mister. Speaking of which, an oil mister is an excellent way to keep your food from sticking to the pan and add some earthy flavor without overdosing on calories and fat; simply pour some extra-virgin olive oil into the mister and use just a spray to coat your pan before cooking.

Window-sill herb garden. You'll have fresh basil, rosemary, thyme, and more right at hand.

A good set of knives. Keep them sharp so slicing and dicing seem like less of a chore.

Colander. For washing produce.

Stackable microwave-safe dishware with lids. To store, pack, and reheat food.

BPA-free water bottle. So you'll always have water close at hand; choose one that's BPA-free (BPA, or *Bisphenol A*, is a chemical that has been linked to infertility, cancer, and weight gain)—avoid bottles with the number "7" in the recycle symbol on the bottom, a sign that it likely contains BPA.

Travel mug. For your green tea.

Load it Up _____

Zero-Calorie Flavor Boosters

Sugar and salt coat your taste buds, masking food's authentic flavor. When you eat clean, however, you can taste what food is *truly* supposed to taste like—maybe for the first time in your adult life! But that doesn't mean you can't still spice things up! Check out all of the calorie-, fat-, salt-, and sugar-free ways you can amp up the flavor. The more adventurous and inventive you are, the better.

VINEGARS

Rice wine vinegar. These can range from sweet and mild to savory. Try it in stir-fries or drizzled on fish and vegetables.

Balsamic vinegar. Splash this over salads or steamed vegetables for flavor and tang—no need for oily dressings! You can also place some in a small saucepan; bring it to a boil, reduce to simmer for about thirty minutes until it has reduced by about half for a thickened, more intense version and then drizzle over asparagus or chicken. (The best way to determine if the reduced vinegar is thick enough is to immerse a metal spoon into the liquid. If it runs right off like water, it's not thick enough; if it clings to the spoon, it's ready.)

Red wine vinegar. This is great in marinades for beef and vegetables.

CITRUS

You can squeeze lemon over practically anything, from steamed broccoli to grilled fish. Or slice up an orange, some lemons, and limes and throw them in a pitcher of water to keep in your refrigerator. It's like having a spa in your kitchen.

MUSTARD

Zero calories, tons of powerful flavor.

GARLIC

Add some garlicky goodness to roasted veggies, chicken, and seafood. But beware: you may sweat it out during cardio tomorrow morning!

HERBS

Basil and oregano. Impart an Italian vibe to steamed or roasted vegetables, fresh tomatoes, chicken, or rice.

Chili powder. A blend of spices—usually chili peppers, onion, garlic, oregano, paprika, and even cinnamon—that kicks up chicken and fish.

Cilantro. This leafy green herb works well with Mexican flavors. Add to salads, vegetables, or meat.

Cumin. An ingredient in most curry powders, this savory spice is nice on chicken, lamb, fish, rice, beans, and vegetables.

Curry blend. Experiment with warm Indian flavors—a curry blend typically includes cumin, turmeric, coriander, chili pepper, mustard, cardamom, ginger, cloves, nutmeg, red pepper, cinnamon, black pepper, and saffron.

Dill. Delicious and tangy on tuna fish, seafood, and green vegetables.

Garlic powder (not garlic salt). Extremely versatile, shake it on steamed or roasted vegetables, chicken, fish, and beef.

Ginger. Gives chicken, seafood, or rice a spicy zing.

Paprika. Lends a deep smoky flavor and beautiful dark red color to chicken, egg, or bean dishes.

Rosemary. Delicious on steamed or roasted vegetables, chicken, fish, or steak.

Thyme. Use this fragrant spice on vegetables, chicken, fish, beef, eggs, and beans.

GET COOKING

The right cooking techniques can make or break your diet, adding in (or helping you avoid) hundreds of potential calories and grams of fat at a single meal. For instance, just two measly tablespoons of oil add 28 grams of fat and more than 240 calories—about the same as a Snickers bar ... and I guarantee your sautéed chicken doesn't taste nearly as good as that chocolaty peanut nougat. Learning to cook with healthier methods like grilling, steaming, poaching, and baking will save you a potential meal's worth of calories without sacrificing flavor.

Method	How it works	Good for
Grilling	Grilling exposes food to an open flame, allowing fat to drip away.	Seafood, poultry, lean meats, vegetables
Baking and roasting	Baking and roasting utilize the high temperature and dry heat inside your oven to cook the food. You may want to place a roasting rack inside the roasting pan to allow fat to drip away.	Seafood, poultry, lean meats, vegetables
Stir-fry	Stir-frying is a traditional Asian method in which small bites of food are quickly cooked in a wok with a very small amount of oil or cooking spray.	Seafood, poultry, lean meats, vegetables
Steaming	Steaming involves placing food inside a perforated basket and hanging it above boiling water. You can also steam food in the microwave.	Vegetables, fish

Cooking Methods or Descriptions to Avoid

When eating out, steer clear of anything labeled fried, deep-fried, sautéed, creamy, breaded, tender, smothered, battered, buttered, al forno, crispy, or loaded. I guarantee it's a bomb of calories, fat, salt, sugar, and cholesterol just waiting to detonate once swallowed.

GROCERY SHOPPING TIPS

All grocery stores are set up the same way: packaged, shelf-stable food goes in the center and fresh produce, meats, dairy, and eggs are stocked along the perimeter. You won't find cookies close to the carrots, and chicken breasts are sold far away from the candy bars. Do yourself a favor: when you go shopping for the week, stick to the perimeter. Fill your cart with fresh and frozen vegetables, lean meats, and egg whites. Then venture to the inner aisles for clean carbs as well as low-calorie, low-fat flavor enhancers like vinegars and spices. Try to fill your cart with produce that is in season, when it's cheaper and more nutrient dense. If you live near a farmer's market, walk to it and treat yourself to some fresh produce.

What to Eat, When

Spring: artichokes, asparagus, green beans, radishes, snap peas, spinach
Summer: beets, bell peppers, berries, cucumbers, eggplant, summer squash, tomatoes, zucchini
Fall: broccoli, brussels sprouts, butternut squash, cauliflower, leeks, mushrooms, sweet potatoes (and apples and pears when in the Maintenance Phase)
Winter: acorn squash, cabbage, collard greens, kale, parsnips, radicchio, turnips (and citrus fruits when in the Maintenance Phase)

HOW TO READ A LABEL

On KO-90 I'd rather you eat whole, natural foods that don't even come with labels. But I'm also a realist, and I understand that most people, once they've lost their weight, will choose to supplement their home cooking with a handful of packaged products. I also realize that our fast-paced lives sometimes mean that we simply don't have time to cook and need quick options. Rather than wander the aisles aimlessly, educate yourself on reading and deciphering labels so you can figure out if an item contains too much sugar, fat, sodium, or calories. Knowledge is a valuable weapon against obesity, paving the way for smart decisions.

First, a little basic math:

Protein and carbohydrates each contain 4 calories per gram.

Fat contains 9 calories per gram.

So if, say, a granola bar contains 150 calories and 6 grams of fat and 3 grams of protein, you can get a quick snapshot of how many of those calories are healthy (from protein) and how many are detrimental (from fat):

6 grams of fat X 9 calories/gram = 54 calories. This means that 54 out of the 150 calories are from fat, or more than one-third of the bar.

3 grams of protein X 4 calories/gram = 12 calories. This means that 12 out of the 150 calories are from protein.

Now, let's take a look at a typical nutrition label and break it down to the essentials:

Nutrition Facts

Serving Size 1 Bar (62g)
Servings Per Container 1

Amount Per Serving

Calories 170   Calories from Fat 80

% Daily Value*

Total Fat 9g	14 %
Saturated Fat 4g	20 %
Trans Fat 0g	
Cholesterol 10mg	3 %
Sodium 55mg	2 %
Total Carbohydrate 22g	7 %
Dietary Fiber less than 1g	3 %
Sugars 18g	
Protein 2g	3 %

Vitamin A	Vitamin C	Calcium	Iron
2 %	6 %	4 %	0 %

Servings per package. First, check the number of servings in the package. If the bag of chips says "3 servings," but you normally eat the whole thing in one sitting, then you have to multiply everything—calories, fat, sodium—by three to determine your intake. In the case of this bar, a serving size is one bar. If you're used to eating two, it's time to scale way back.

Calories from fat. Pay particular attention to the "Calories from fat" figure: if a serving of macaroni and cheese contains 260 calories per serving, and 120 calories are from fat, that means nearly half of the calories in a single serving come from fat. In the case of this bar, 80 out of 170 calories, or nearly half, are from fat.

Saturated fat. Stick to less than one gram per serving.

Trans fat. Avoid these completely, as they increase the risk of coronary heart disease by elevating levels of LDL ("bad") cholesterol and reducing levels of HDL ("good") cholesterol.

Total carbohydrate. Stick to less than 30 grams per serving. The Total Carbohydrate section is further broken down into Dietary fiber and Sugars. For the former, choose options that will help you reach a total of 15 to 30 grams per day. Under "Sugars," aim for no more than 5 percent of your total daily carbohydrate content per serving. For example, if you consume 150 grams of carbs per day on KO-90, you would want the label to list no more than 7.5 grams of sugar.

Cholesterol. Stick to less than 20 mg per serving.

* Percent Daily Values are based on a 2,000 calorie diet. Your Daily Values may be higher or lower depending on your calorie needs.

	Calories:	2,000	2,500
Total Fat	Less than	65g	80g
Sat Fat	Less than	20g	25g
Cholesterol	Less than	300mg	300mg
Sodium	Less than	2,400mg	2,400mg
Total Carbohydrate		300g	375g
Dietary Fiber		25g	30g

Sodium. Stick to less than 140 mg per serving.

Most food labels will tell you—usually at the bottom—that "**Percent Daily Values are based on a 2,000 calorie diet.**" The portion of the label doesn't change from item to item—it's the same on a box of brown sugar as a bag of Doritos. Pay attention.

Look at the amounts listed in the 2,000-calorie column; these are the Daily Values (DV), or recommended levels of intakes, for each nutrient. Make a concerted effort to keep your daily intake within these parameters, physically tallying up your foods and amounts as you progress through the day. (Eventually you'll be able to keep track mentally, but for now it's far more accurate to write it down. Bonus: research proves that logging your meals and snacks helps significantly with weight loss and maintenance.)

AVOID PORTION DISTORTION

Portion sizes have ballooned in recent years, to the point at which a single restaurant portion of pasta is enough to feed a family of four. In the past twenty years the average plate of spaghetti and meatballs has mushroomed from 500 calories (one cup of pasta with sauce plus three small meatballs) to 1,025 calories (two cups of pasta with sauce plus three large meatballs). A chicken Caesar salad now weighs in at 790 calories (3.5 cups) versus the 390 calories (1.5 cups) it was at previously. Even something as simple as coffee, which is calorie-free, now packs more fat and calories than multiple candy bars, thanks to whipped cream, caramel drizzles, and whole milk.[10]

_____ It's in the Bag **PJ's**
Pointer

Buy yourself one or two refrigerated, insulated bags and reusable ice packs and then stash them in your kitchen. You can use them to tote healthy, home-prepared lunches to work, where your food will stay cold and fresh.

With that in mind, it's essential that you retrain your brain to recognize—and feel satisfied on—normal portion sizes. Keep the following comparisons in mind, especially while dining out:

1 cup of cereal = a fist
1/2 cup of cooked rice = 1/2 baseball
1 baked sweet potato = a computer mouse
3 ounces fish, chicken, or lean beef = the palm of your hand (minus the fingers and thumb)
2 tablespoons of peanut butter = a Ping-Pong ball
1 medium fruit = a baseball (Maintenance Phase only)
1/2 cup of fresh fruit = 1/2 baseball (Maintenance Phase only)
1 1/2 ounces of low-fat or fat-free cheese = 4 stacked dice (Maintenance Phase only)
1/2 cup of ice cream = 1/2 baseball (Maintenance Phase only)

SUPPLEMENTS

Supplements act like health insurance, guaranteeing that you don't fall short on key nutrients. I advise my clients to take the same supplements I take myself:

(Of course, as with any plan, be sure to check with your health care provider before starting a new supplement regimen in order to prevent any potential drug interactions.)

Vitamin C (calcium ascorbate). 1000 mg twice a day

Why: Vitamin C is a building block for collagen, a protein used to inject skin with elasticity and form tendons, ligaments, blood vessels, and scar tissue. It assists with the growth and repair of tissues throughout your body and promotes wound healing. Vitamin C is also a powerful antioxidant and immune-system enhancer.

Barley grass tablets. Two in the morning and two in the afternoon

Why: Similar to wheatgrass, barley grass helps to reduce system-wide inflammation and pain, making it a great workout recovery tool. It also keeps your body's pH levels balanced (years of sugary, fatty junk food has likely tipped your system to an acidic state; an alkaline system is a pro-fat-loss system. You can purchase these at your local natural health food store.

Flaxseed oil. 1000 mg three times a day

Why: Rich in heart-healthy omega-3 fatty acids, flaxseed oil has been shown to reduce inflammation and cholesterol and help prevent chronic diseases such as heart disease and arthritis. I recommend a half teaspoon of flaxseed oil (or two liquid capsules) three times a day. Alternatively, you can drizzle a half teaspoon over your salad along with balsamic vinegar.

Calcium. 500 mg twice a day

Why: Because dairy is limited during the first three months of this plan (and possibly longer), shoring up on bone-building calcium is important. Be sure to choose a brand with Vitamin D: if calcium is the "bricks" of your skeleton, Vitamin D is the mortar.

Calcium has also been shown to play a role in fat loss. A landmark University of Tennessee-Knoxville study found that individuals who consumed 1,100 mg of calcium per day lost 22 percent more weight and 61 percent more body fat than those who only ate 500 mg of calcium per day.[11]

Potassium. 100 mg twice a day

Why: This mineral helps regulate blood pressure, and deficient levels of potassium have been linked with heart disease, stroke, arthritis, and cancer. It also helps restore alkalinity. (See PJ's Pointer, "Acid versus Alkaline," below.) If you've been diagnosed with diabetes or heart disease, check with your doctor before taking potassium.

During especially heavy workouts, add:

Magnesium. 420 mg a day for men; 320 mg a day for women

Why: Magnesium helps maintain normal muscle and nerve function, supports a healthy immune system, and may help asthmatics to breathe easier.[12]

Acid versus Alkaline PJ's Pointer

When we eat poorly—soda, fried foods, red meat—our body recognizes the foods as acidic and attempts to protect itself. That's because acid can be corrosive and, over time, may damage organs and cause deterioration. In defense the body builds up a protective anti-acid layer of fat. That's why many people carry weight in their midsection, hips, and chest; those spots are in closest proximity to our major organs. When we start fueling ourselves with vegetables and whole grains—alkaline foods—we rebalance the body's pH levels and send the message that it no longer needs to store fat for protection. The result: a leaner chest area, slimmer waistline, narrower hips, and a happier, healthier heart.

CAFFEINE

A hit of caffeine can help power you through a workout, especially if you're waking up early in the morning. But too many of us are addicted to the artificial jolt, and too much caffeine will compromise your sleep. If so, the repercussions extend beyond just getting drowsy in a work meeting: sleep is a vital regulator of body weight and metabolism. Just a few nights of tossing and turning can cause levels of hunger-regulating hormone leptin to plummet, while ghrelin, another hormone that increases appetite, rises. In one Stanford University/University of Wisconsin study of one thousand volunteers, those who slept fewer than eight hours a night had higher body-fat percentages, and those who clocked the least shut-eye weighed the most.[13]

If you must drink coffee, keep it to one to two cups per day, drink it black with no milk or sugar, and don't consume it late at night. Caffeine-free herbal teas are a smarter option because they contain high concentrations of antioxidants. Feel free to drink as many cups as you like. And be prepared not to *need* as much caffeine: Your morning workouts will naturally hike up your energy level and boost your mood.

THE JAPANESE WAY OF EATING

Being based in Asia for seven years I fell in love with Asian food. I'm not talking about the greasy Chinese food you can get at the mall, like oily Kung Pao Chicken or fried rice; I mean authentic Japanese cuisine: sushi, sashimi, rice, and exotic vegetables. There's a reason the Japanese have such long life expectancies and low rates of obesity: they eat clean, without much added fat or sugar (one exception is salt: miso soup and soy sauce are extremely high in sodium). Furthermore, they stick to small portions, eat slowly and mindfully, and walk everywhere. Need more proof of how dismal America's diet is? When Japanese people move to the United States and adopt Western eating habits, they gain weight, increase their risk of heart disease and cancer, and shorten their life span.

You can enjoy some of the same health and weight benefits as the Japanese do by adopting their dietary and lifestyle habits.

Eat fish—lots of it. An excellent source of lean protein, fish—particularly whitefish varieties such as tilapia, cod, flounder, and mahi mahi—is low in calories and cholesterol. Avoid salmon and other fatty fish until you've progressed to the Maintenance Phase.

Incorporate vegetables as often as possible. Traditional Japanese favorites include shiitake mushrooms, carrots, bamboo shoots, daikon (white radish), eggplant, onions, bell peppers, and seaweed/other sea vegetables.

Cook lightly. Most meals are prepared without a heavy amount of oil or butter. Vegetables and meats are often steamed, stir-fried in a small amount of oil, or simmered in broth.

Keep portions small. Avoid swallowing huge bites of food. Research shows that when we're served more, we tend to eat it—whether we planned to and were hungry for it or not. People eat up to 45 percent more food when served bigger helpings, scientists from the University of Illinois, Urbana-Champaign report.

Replace bread with rice. Rice is a low-fat complex carbohydrate that offers belly-filling fiber and magnesium, which is necessary for healthy muscle and nerve functioning.

The Japanese enjoy their rice plain, without butter. And watch your serving size: one cup—the amount you could fit inside a baseball—contains about two hundred calories.

Stop when you're full. The Japanese don't wolf down food in front of the computer or eat while standing up in front of the fridge. They treat their food with more respect, chewing slowly and mindfully. They also practice a theory known as *hara hachi bu*, which means eat until you are 80 percent full. Stop before your stomach starts to grow uncomfortable and let your body catch up with your mouth. It takes time—around twenty minutes—for your mind to register fullness.

Drink green tea. A mainstay in Japanese culture, I sip decaffeinated green tea all day long. It's credited with contributing to Japan's low rates of cancer and heart disease. Newer studies have also suggested that the hot drink may help burn fat, prevent diabetes, and even thwart dementia.[14]

DIET FOODS THAT AREN'T

It's amazing how many people will order a large raisin-bran muffin, a lite yogurt, and a skinny latte for breakfast and think they're helping themselves to achieve a healthy weight. They simply don't realize that more than a thousand calories, plus plenty of sugar and fat, are hidden inside. Consumers have been brainwashed to think that anything with the word "diet" or "lite" in it is good for them, including diet soda, lite ice cream, diet salad

---

SHOW ME THE SCIENCE

Go Whole or Go Home

When it comes to shedding weight, whole grains trump refined carbs every time. In a twelve-year study following nearly seventy-five thousand female nurses, weight was consistently lower among those women who consumed more whole grains.[15]

Whole grains can also:

- lower your heart disease risk,[16]
- help prevent weight gain, and[17]
- slash diabetes risk.[18]

---

dressing, and more. Then there are foods that *seem* like they'd be kind to your waistline but are actually just covert junk food. Here's what you should avoid:

Granola and granola bars. Those hearty oats and grains are coated in butter or even fried before they get mixed with high-sugar dried fruit and stamped with a "Good for You!" label.

Juice and bottled tea. Unless the tea is unsweetened, it's loaded with sugary calories. Same thing goes for juice.

Diet soda. It's no secret that sugary sodas contribute to obesity. In fact, drinking just one soda a day will result in a weight gain of two pounds of pure fat within a year. But research suggests that diet soda is no good either; artificial sugars may actually *stimulate* your appetite. Pour 'em out.

Low-fat yogurt. "Low fat" usually means "high sugar." An average cup of low-fat fruit-on-the-bottom yogurt is loaded with six teaspoons of added sugar.

Deli meat. Besides sky-high sodium levels, consumption of processed meat has been linked to stomach cancer.

Salads. Actually, salads are fantastic. It's the dressing that gets ladled over them that will derail you. Most commercial dressings are loaded with fats, oils, preservatives as well as sodium and high-fructose corn syrup. Go naked with your greens or adorn them simply with vinegar and oil. Ditto for cheese, bacon bits, croutons, and pasta salads—these additions will derail you faster than you can say, "I'll have the chopped chicken salad, please."

Muffins. These are nothing but massive cupcakes without the frosting. Packed with white flour, butter, oil, and sugar, even a seemingly saintly bran muffin studded with raisins can pack five hundred calories—more than a third of your daily needs!

Smoothies and frozen yogurt. You could spend forty-five minutes on the treadmill and—Poof!—erase all of your hard work with a few gulps. A Banana Berry Power Smoothie from Jamba Juice packs 560 calories and 115 grams of sugar.

Bagels. AKA carb bombs—high in calories with little nutritional benefit.

Sushi. Having lived in Japan, I'm a huge fan of sushi and sashimi done right. But done wrong, it can handily sabotage your efforts. A twelve-piece Dragon Roll (eel, cucumbers, avocado, eel sauce, seaweed, and rice) contains more than five hundred calories and eighteen grams of fat. Other sushi bar disasters include spicy tuna (it's mixed with mayonnaise), the Philadelphia Roll (cream cheese), and anything with the word "tempura" in the description. These aren't traditional maki rolls but rather Americanized versions. Stick to basic fish, rice, and seaweed.

Low-carb beer. It's still just liquid calories with no nutritive value.

Your KO-90 Cheat Sheet

Eat clean.
Load up on vegetables and lean protein.
Drink your protein shakes.
Stay hydrated.
Avoid dairy.
Stick to the plan.
Use an olive oil mister and bake, grill, or steam your hot meals.
Reach for herbs for fantastic flavor, not the salt shaker.
Skip the artificial sweeteners and "diet" products.
Shop the perimeter of your grocery store.
Avoid caffeine at night—or entirely, if possible.
Eat like the person you wish to become, not the person you are now. It *will* get easier.

MAINTENANCE PLAN

The seven-day KO-90 Jumpstart should be repeated for the first three months. Feel free to exchange breakfasts with other breakfasts, lunches with other lunches, and dinners with other dinners to change things up and keep your palate surprised. Once you've reached your target weight (or are within about five to ten pounds of it), it's time to switch to the Maintenance Plan. That means it's time to start reintroducing reasonable portions of healthy foods that you've been missing or craving. You deserve it! Plus, by this point your body will have transformed internally as well as externally, so your metabolism can handle an increase in nutritious calories. And to be honest, not every new food needs to be entirely wholesome; once you're within close range of your target weight, even foods you might consider "bad," like pasta, pizza, or fries, can still have a place in an overall healthy eating plan. At this point it's about portion control: enjoying a small amount of your treat of choice (one bowl of pasta, one slice of pizza, one small container of fries), bumping up your evening walk from fifteen to thirty minutes, and moving on.

But as I've mentioned repeatedly throughout the book, my bet is that you'll be so encouraged by your progress that you'll want to keep eating clean. You'll remember how sluggish and bloated fast food used to make you feel, how uncomfortable that post-pizza food coma felt. In that case you might want to stick with adding in more traditionally healthy foods that aren't included in the Jumpstart Plan, such as low-fat dairy, fruit, nuts, healthy fats, and so forth. Here's an example of what a day on the Maintenance Plan might look like (I've bolded the possible changes):

Breakfast

3.5 large shredded-wheat biscuits sprinkled with 1.8 ounces protein powder, mixed with **7 ounces of skim, 1 percent, or 2 percent milk and topped with a quarter cup mixed berries**. Serve with one cup of black coffee.

Morning Snack

One cup 2 percent Greek yogurt mixed with 1 tablespoon honey *or* a small handful of almonds.

Lunch

Tuna salad: 5 ounces spring water–packed tuna, 1.5 ounces each tomato, cucumber, and celery, as much lettuce as you like, and one teaspoon balsamic vinegar, **enjoy as an open-faced sandwich on a slice of whole wheat bread. Half a cup of "spiral" pasta can also be added, and balsamic vinegar can be substituted with 1 tablespoon homemade mayonnaise.**

Afternoon Snack

Cut 2.5 hard-boiled eggs in half and season with cracked pepper. Serve with a small handful of celery and carrot sticks (six of each, four inches long).

Late-Afternoon Snack

Mix 1.8 ounces protein powder with 8 ounces water.

Dinner

One 6-ounce white-flesh fish fillet (tilapia, flounder, sea bass), seasoned with herbs, sprinkled with lemon juice, wrapped in aluminum foil, and baked on a tray with a shallow water bath at 350°F for fourteen minutes or until cooked through. Serve with 3.5 ounces sweet potato fries (cut sweet potato into French fry shape or wedges; add whole cloves of garlic and rosemary sprigs and season with cracked pepper, cumin, and a half teaspoon of extra-virgin olive oil; bake on nonstick tray at 400°F for thirty minutes or until crispy and cooked through), 3.5 ounces steamed, mixed vegetables, and **one glass of merlot. Sweet potato fries can be substituted with Coliban potato fries if so desired.**

My suggestion is not to make all of these changes at once; stick to one or two new foods per day. After a few weeks, if your weight is still decreasing (if you are still trying to lose more weight) or remains steady (if you've already reached your goal weight), you're doing everything right. Once again, YOU are in control!

If you make all of these changes in one day, you'll need to up your activity—so stick with one to two changes per day.

True success, as far as I'm concerned, is when someone doesn't have to think about food or weight. But your cravings will be gone—your body will be so clean internally that it won't want junk food. At that point you'll have formed healthy eating habits, you'll understand portion control, and you'll be disciplined with your training.

TIPS TO LIVE BY

By now you can probably see some of my favorite tricks of the trade: I'm a huge fan of protein and veggies, I don't want you skipping breakfast, and water is my drink of choice. Below, I've put together a list of some of my other best tips to keep you fresh, fueled, and far from famished:

- At the beginning of the week prepare about a dozen lean turkey roll-ups: layer cucumbers and bell pepper slices with lean, thinly sliced meat and then roll them up like little cigars. Stash them in the fridge for a quick and hearty snack.
- Also at the start of the week cook up a batch of sweet potatoes. I like to wash and wrap them in foil and bake them at 400°F for fifteen to twenty minutes; you'll know they're ready when a toothpick or knife cleanly slips in and out of the middle of the potato. The spuds will last for about a week in the fridge or up to a month in the freezer.
- Buy an oil mister. There's a reason I included it in my list of Healthy Kitchen Tools—everyone should own one. They're inexpensive (I bought mine for less than

$20) and will prevent your food from sticking to the pan—and your glutes. That's because you get a hint of earthy flavor without overdosing on calories and fat. Simply pour some extra-virgin olive oil into the mister and use just a spray to coat your pan before cooking, your vegetables before roasting, or your fish before baking. It will also help your bottle of olive oil last ten times as long as pouring would.

- Keep a large pitcher of water in your fridge, but spice it up with sliced lemon, lime, cucumber, or even sprigs of fresh mint. It's like spa water in your own kitchen! I also like to keep two large, one-liter bottles of water in the fridge at all times, making sure I drink both of them by the end of the day.

PANTRY LIST

Keep yourself on track with a pantry stocked with the following KO-90 staples:

Oatmeal
Protein powder
Cans of tuna fish (spring water–packed)
Wasa Crisps
Rice
Sweet potatoes
Onions
Garlic
Flaxseed oil
Olive oil spray
Balsamic and assorted other vinegars
Herbs and spices
Tea and/or coffee
Vitamins and supplements
And LOTS of leafy greens

PART 5

GET THE LEAD OUT

Move Your Body

Now it's time for you to experience what I learned in that Tokyo gym twelve years ago: with a carefully crafted plan, the right know-how, and the same amount of time you typically spend watching bad late-night TV, you can ditch the fat and carve out a new masterpiece of a physique. I've already taken care of the first and second requirements, so all you need to do is show up. First of all, know this:

What you know or have been told about exercising is probably mostly wrong.

A huge amount of misinformation exists about exercise. You do not need to work out as if you were a contestant on a weight-loss reality show in order to slim down in an efficient manner. KO-90 is all about maximizing your time in the gym and using your workouts to enhance your newly revamped eating habits. Here are a few exercise myths I hear from clients all the time:

IF THIRTY MINUTES OF CARDIO A DAY IS GOOD, AN HOUR A DAY IS BETTER.

There's absolutely no need to spend hours a day training as if you were a professional athlete. In fact, too much cardio will prove counterproductive: after about thirty minutes you'll begin burning muscle if you're not careful. But our goal is to torch *fat*. Limiting cardio to fifteen minutes in the morning and another fifteen at night makes it manageable and easy to fit into a packed schedule, plus it allows you to really go full force with purpose rather than speed when you are working out, burning as much fat as possible.

I NEED TO FUEL UP BEFORE CARDIO.

Marathon runners need to carbo load before a race, but you do not. By waking up and working out on an empty stomach you're forcing your body to use its fat stores for fuel. However, if you eat a meal immediately beforehand, you'll just be working off those calories instead of the fat stores. When you exercise before breakfast, you start your day off with a calorie deficit—you've burned more than you've taken in. It's fantastic for putting you in a healthy mindset and will subconsciously guide your eating decisions all day long.

THE MORE AB EXERCISES I DO, THE FLATTER MY STOMACH WILL GET.

Abdominal exercises will improve your core strength, but it's really your diet that determines how ripped your stomach appears. Picture your abs as a mattress (the muscles) with a blanket over it (fat and skin.) You might have the firmest mattress on the market, but if you've got a super thick, lumpy blanket lying on top, nobody will ever know. I'm helping you to strip away the blanket. Stick to an every-other-day routine for ab exercises. That's what I do.

I HAVE TO BE IN SHAPE TO JOIN A GYM.

Here's the thing about gyms: most people there feel insecure about their bodies. This goes for the muscle-bound men in the weight room too. The truth is that everyone is so focused on their own bodies that the last thing they're worried about is how *you* look. And I can pretty much guarantee that you'll see people of all shapes and sizes working out—not just slender hard-bodies.

Consider your gym membership an investment in your health. When choosing a facility, look for a wide variety of equipment and a knowledgeable and caring staff. Don't be afraid to ask members about their experiences. Here are some other questions to consider: Does it seem clean? Is there a long wait time for machines? Does the staff look approachable and in shape? I prefer a friendly environment with a noncompetitive vibe, but go with what motivates *you*. Some people like more of a nightclub ambiance; others prefer a more utilitarian feel. You can always shop around—lots of gyms offer trial memberships, free classes, or free initial training sessions. Let them do the hard work for you, helping you find a place that's going to inspire and encourage you.

Wherever you choose, you'll find that having other like-minded individuals around can be highly motivating, and their workouts and determination will inspire you to keep going. Keep in mind that most people are at the gym to take care of their own health and fitness, not to gauge yours!

I DON'T NEED TO JOIN A GYM BECAUSE I CAN DO LUNGES AND SQUATS AT HOME.

It's true that there has been a shift away from gyms, with experts claiming you can get an effective workout at home using moves that utilize your own body weight. But for KO-90 followers, whose goal is to burn fat, build muscle, and tone up simultaneously, a well-stocked gym is absolutely essential. There's no way the average person could afford—or store—the dozens of resistance machines, free weights, and cardio equipment necessary to achieve all three goals. Plus, it's a dedicated facility where you can go with a single purpose in mind—no distractions like the computer, the refrigerator, the phone, or the laundry. It's hard enough to lose weight on your own, so set yourself up for success as much as possible by investing in a quality workout facility.

STRETCHING IS OVERRATED—WHO CARES ABOUT BEING FLEXIBLE?

You should care. The goal is not to be able to do the splits but rather to keep your muscles pliable and prevent injury. No part of your body exists in a vacuum. Tight hamstrings, for example, can cause lower back pain. Stretching relieves the muscular tension that accumulates during your workout and will give you that highly sought-after long, lean look.

With KO-90 you'll stretch between every set. Let's say you just completed ten reps of a chest exercise. You'll stretch your chest muscles immediately after and then move into your second set of strength-training exercises. This maximizes your workout's efficiency, as you don't need to dedicate an extra twenty minutes at the end of your routine to stretching.

A STEADY PACE WINS THE RACE DURING CARDIO.

Just the opposite is true, in fact. Interval training—alternating a faster pace with a moderate one—is proven to kick-start your metabolism and burn more fat. In one recent

KEEP IT OFF

fifteen-week study, subjects who mixed jogging and sprinting for twenty minutes shed three times the fat from their legs and glutes versus those who jogged steadily for forty minutes.[1] Start your cardio with a one-minute warm-up and then alternate a minute at a fast pace with a minute at a more moderate (but not too slow) pace. You should feel as if you're really pushing yourself during the "up" minutes, working at about 80 percent of your maximum heart rate (see Part 2, page 27). During your "down" minutes, shoot for 60 to 65 percent. Initially, you might not be able to talk at all during cardio, but eventually you should still be carry on with short bits of conversation during your "down" minutes. By the same token, don't go flat out for fifteen minutes either; you will just end up burning muscle and your body will look and feel tired. Challenge yourself, but in a sensible fashion. Remember that slower-paced cardio is better than bullet-like speed.

I'M A WOMAN; WEIGHTS WILL BULK ME UP.

Not at all. You need high levels of testosterone to start building bulky muscles. But although you won't have monstrous quads or biceps, you *will* develop great strength, fat-burning capability, and tone.

BENEFITS OF STRENGTH TRAINING

> torches fat and calories
> boosts cardio efficiency and endurance
> prevents injuries and speeds recovery
> builds your bones

SHOW ME THE SCIENCE

A recent study found that a single set of ten strength-training exercises blazes an extra hundred calories per day for *three days* postworkout. That means just fifteen minutes of weights actually burns four hundred–plus calories.[2]

Exercise can be addictive. I've had clients who absolutely hated working out and, prior to seeking my help, had refused to even set foot in a gym. By Week 2 you can't keep them *out* of the gym. They start to feel healthier almost immediately, and they see changes in their body. Emotionally, the feeling of doing something good for yourself will create a high that no potato chip or ice cream could ever make—and the effects snowball. The same will happen for you.

helps your body fight age-related changes by maintaining lean muscle mass

decreases your risk of developing Type 2 diabetes[3]

elevates your mood

improves your posture

truly changes the shape of your body

THE MOVES

The KO-90 plan is simple and doable. You'll kick off every day with fifteen minutes of cardio. On four to five days out of the week you'll hit the gym for a fifty-minute strength-training routine and abdominal work. At night you'll commit to a fifteen-minute walk. You'll have rest days to allow your muscles to recover and grow, but the 15/15 cardio every day is a must.

BEGINNER WORKOUT

This is the routine you will follow until you have lost 70 percent of your total weight-loss goal, at which point you will follow the Advanced Workout. In other words:

If you want to lose a hundred pounds, follow the Beginner Workout until you've lost seventy pounds.

If you want to lose seventy-five pounds, follow the Beginner Workout until you've lost fifty-three pounds.

SUCCESS STORY DORA

"I had tried medication to deal with my depression and anxiety—it didn't work very well. But once I started training with PJ, I discovered that exercise gives your body the chemicals it needs to feel better. Exercise became fun—I actually love to go to the gym now. My sleep apnea is gone, my blood pressure normalized. Despite the fact that meal delivery service, women-only gyms, and even gastric bypass had failed, PJ gave me the tools to shrink from a size 30 to a size 6."

—Dora Dogas, age thirty-five, lost 198 pounds . . . and counting

"I struggled with the eating plan for the first month, but with PJ's ongoing support I was able to stick it out, and it has given me a new lifestyle, helped my relationship—my wife is also a client—and changed the way I look at what foods are good to eat and what to stay away from. I am so happy with the way I look; my original goal weight was 209 pounds, but with PJ's help I have smashed that down to 205 and 7 percent body fat!"

—**Hutch Saluni,** age thirty-two, lost 32 pounds

If you want to lose fifty pounds, follow the Beginner Workout until you've lost thirty-five pounds.

If you want to lose twenty-five pounds, follow the Beginner Workout until you've lost eighteen pounds.

The Beginner Workout includes four weekly weight sessions, alternating between upper and lower body and none lasting more than fifty minutes. Strive for two days on, followed by a rest day, then another two days on, followed by two more rest days. Abdominal work will accompany cardio every other morning. As for cardio, I want you to commit to fifteen minutes every morning on an empty stomach. In the evening let your food digest for forty-five minutes after dinner and then work in another fifteen minutes of brisk walking.

A typical week will look like this:

	Monday	Tuesday	Wednesday	Thursday	Friday	Saturday	Sunday
7 a.m.	15 minutes of cardio	15 minutes of cardio	15 minutes of cardio	15 minutes of cardio	15 minutes of cardio	15 minutes of cardio	15 minutes of cardio
	Abs		Abs		Abs		Abs
5 p.m.	Upper-body weights	Lower-body weights		Upper-body weights	Lower-body weights		
Evening	15-minute walk	15-minute walk	15-minute walk	15-minute walk	15-minute walk	15-minute walk	15-minute walk

Monday: morning cardio and abs, evening upper-body weights, evening cardio
Tuesday: morning cardio, evening lower-body weights, evening cardio
Wednesday: morning cardio and abs, evening cardio, no weights
Thursday: morning cardio, evening upper-body weights, evening cardio
Friday: morning cardio and abs, evening lower-body weights, evening cardio
Saturday: morning and evening cardio, no weights or abs
Sunday: morning cardio and abs, evening cardio, no weights

Although changing the order of the exercises is fine, don't skip any. I know it's easy to say, "Ditching Glute Kickbacks today won't make a difference"—especially if you happen to hate Glute Kickbacks! But before you know it you'll start skipping two moves, then three, and you'll get nowhere, fast. I thought I could cut corners when I first started working out again, and payback came in the form of a scale that wouldn't budge and clothes that weren't getting any looser. Not until I followed exactly what I preached to my clients did I start to see a real difference . . . and look at me now!

In the beginning you will complete a single twelve-set rep for each upper-body exercise and a single fifteen-set rep for each lower-body exercise. After about ten sessions you should be able to bump that up to two sets each and, soon thereafter, three sets each for maximum results.

As far as weight is concerned, it's much smarter to start at a lower level and increase rather than attempt to lift something too heavy and risk injuring yourself. Always begin on the lightest weight and add small increments of two to five pounds as your body and confidence grow stronger. That said, if the lightest weight feels *so* light you can barely feel it, move up a few notches so it becomes challenging, but not impossible. With free weights start with three- or five-pound dumbbells. With any sort of exercise calling for a bar, perform the move first with no weights on the bar. Most cable machines will automatically start at ten pounds.

If your gym doesn't have the specific piece of equipment mentioned, ask a staff member to show you an alternative move. You can feel free to play around with the order of exercises, but each one should be performed, increasing the weight for each set when possible. The first set of reps for each move should feel moderately difficult, the second set should feel challenging, and the final round should feel tough. Rest thirty seconds between sets but not more than that (this is not the time to start flipping through a magazine or chatting with a neighbor—both will derail you).

SUCCESS STORY **BERNADETTE**

"My arms are now cut and my legs are slim and tight. Lifting weights has also given me great posture. I see the same results in PJ's other clients. You don't just lose weight; you lose fat—and that looks fantastic on women."
—**Bernadette Clarebrough**, age fifty-one, lost 53 pounds

Much like your morning cardio, you want to lift weights without a pile of food in your stomach. Refrain from eating for about one hour to ninety minutes before your workout to avoid feeling sluggish or causing cramps. Re-fuel after your workout.

Upper Body (three sets of twelve reps each)

BARBELL BENCH PRESS

Primary muscles worked: **Pectoralis major (chest)**
Secondary muscles worked: **Deltoids (shoulders), triceps, biceps**

Lie down on a flat bench and grasp Olympic (straight) bar with overhead hands and a wide grip. Push up slightly to dismount the bar and lower weight so that it just touches your chest. Press upward until arms are fully extended (do not allow elbows to lock). Repeat twelve times.

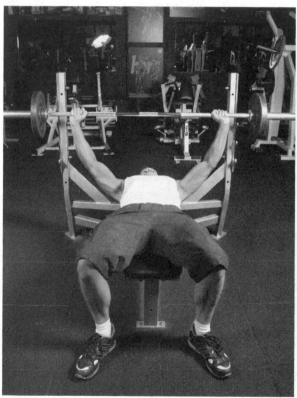 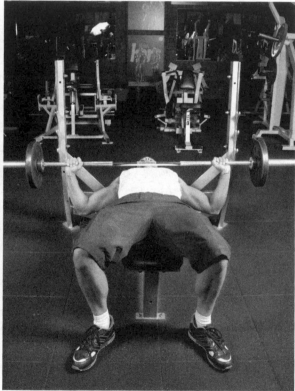

SEATED PEC DECK

Primary muscles worked: **Pectoralis major, pectoralis minor (chest)**
Secondary muscles worked: **Deltoids (shoulders)**

Sit down with your back facing the pad. Reaching back one arm at a time, grip handles on either side. Squeeze your clenched fists together so that they nearly touch (but don't actually touch) in front of you. Slowly return to the starting position. Repeat twelve times.

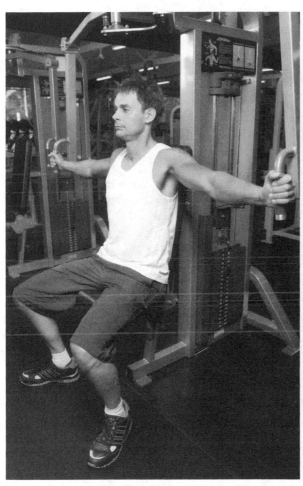 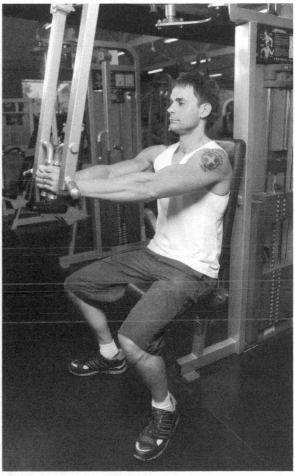

REVERSE CABLE CROSSOVERS

Primary muscles worked: **Posterior deltoid (shoulders), rhomboids (upper back), trapezius (upper back)**

Secondary muscles worked: **Latissimus dorsi (back)**

Stand in the center of the cable crossover machine with soft knees and a contracted core. Making sure the handles of the pulleys are in the uppermost position, grasp them with opposite hands (your arms will be crossed in front of you). Pull handles across and back, starting and finishing at midback level and hyperextending without bending your elbows, and slowly return to where your hands are crossed in front of you. Repeat twelve times.

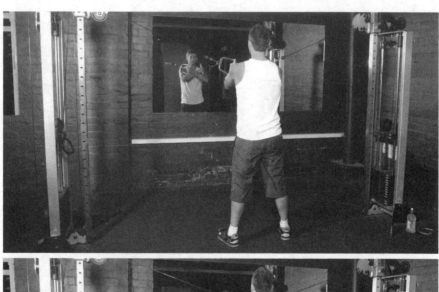

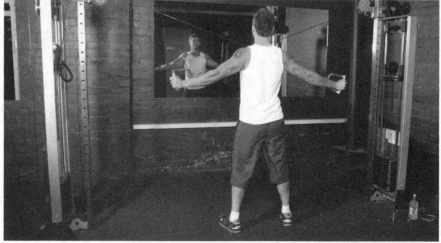

INCLINE SHOULDER PRESS

Primary muscles worked: **Deltoids (shoulders), triceps, trapezius (upper back)**

Secondary muscles worked: **Rhomboids (upper back), teres major (back/shoulder), teres minor (back/shoulder)**

Sit down and reach back to grasp handles, holding them above each shoulder with elbows pointing down. Push upward until arms are extended overhead (do not allow elbows to lock). Return to starting position. Repeat twelve times.

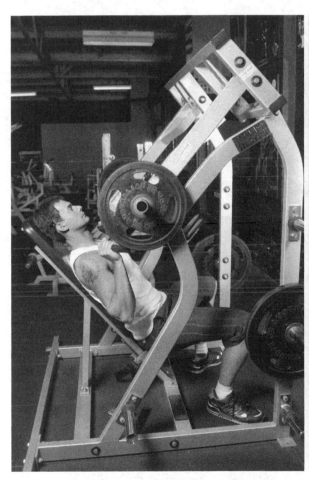 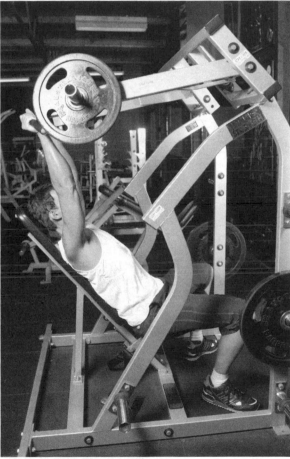

DUMBBELL FRONT RAISES

Muscles worked: **Deltoids (shoulders)**

Standing with feet apart, grasp a dumbbell in each hand, palms facing down, slightly in front of upper legs, with elbows slightly bent. One at a time, raise each arm up and out in front of you until it is parallel with the floor. Slowly return to starting position. Repeat twelve times per side.

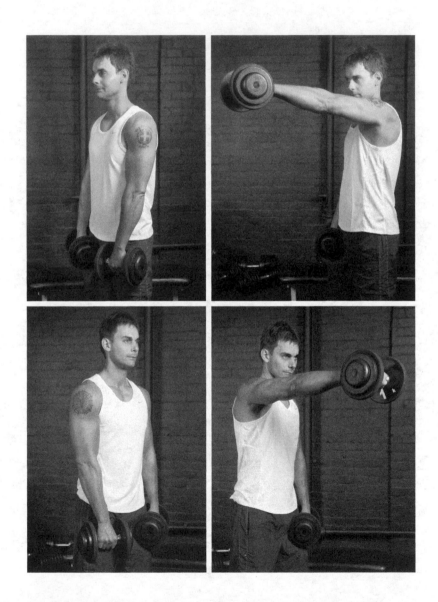

DUMBBELL SHRUGS

Muscles worked: **Upper trapezius, middle trapezius, levator scapulae (all back)**

In a standing position with feet apart, holding a dumbbell in each hand, shrug shoulders as high as possible, then lower. Repeat twelve times.

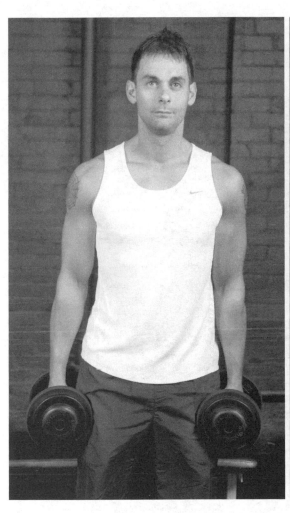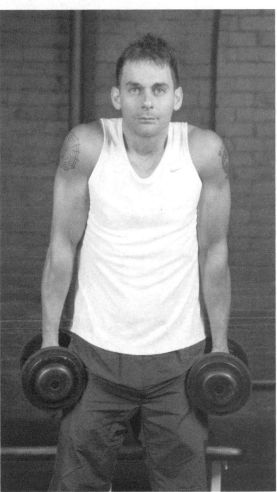

EZ BAR STANDING BICEP CURLS

Muscles worked: **Biceps**

Standing straight with feet apart and a soft bend in the knees, hold the EZ bar in your hands, arms slightly bent with palms up and wider than shoulder width apart. Keeping your elbows tucked in, raise your forearms until your elbows are completely flexed and your forearms are touching your biceps. Return to starting position. Repeat twelve times.

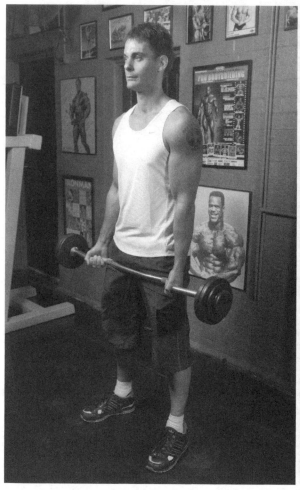
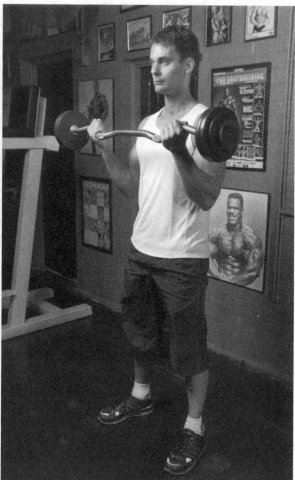

OVERHEAD ROPE EXTENSIONS

Muscles worked: **Triceps brachii (triceps)**

Stand with your back to a high pulley and reach overhead with the rope in your hand. Take one step forward to elevate the weight stack. Keeping your back straight and hips slightly forward, with your thumbs above your head and elbows facing straight ahead, extend arms until fully extended and then twist the rope so that palms face the ground. Slowly allow arms to bend back to starting position. Repeat twelve times.

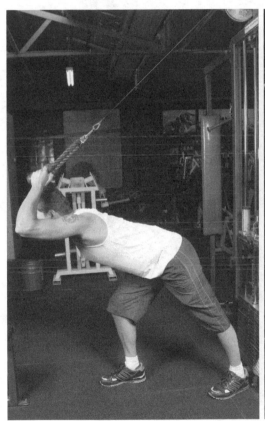 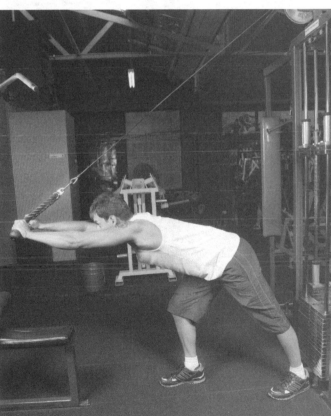

SEATED INCLINE DUMBBELL CURL

Muscles worked: **Biceps brachii, brachialis, brachioradialis (biceps)**

Adjust an incline bench between 45 and 60 degrees. Holding a dumbbell in each hand, sit down, lie back, and lower arms so they are hanging straight toward the floor (palms facing forward). In a controlled fashion begin curling, alternating between left and right arms, making sure to keep elbows close to your body. Repeat twelve times per side.

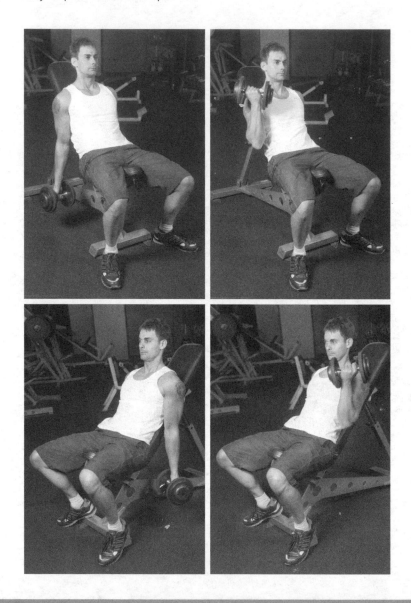

TRICEPS PUSHDOWNS

Muscles worked: **Triceps brachii (triceps)**

Stand facing a high pulley with a straight bar or V bar. Grip the bar, palms down, a bit narrower than shoulder width and bring the bar down so your elbows are close to your body, and your forearms, when parallel to the floor, are waist level. Continue pushing down until your arms are nearly extended. Pause for two seconds then return forearms to waist level. Repeat twelve times.

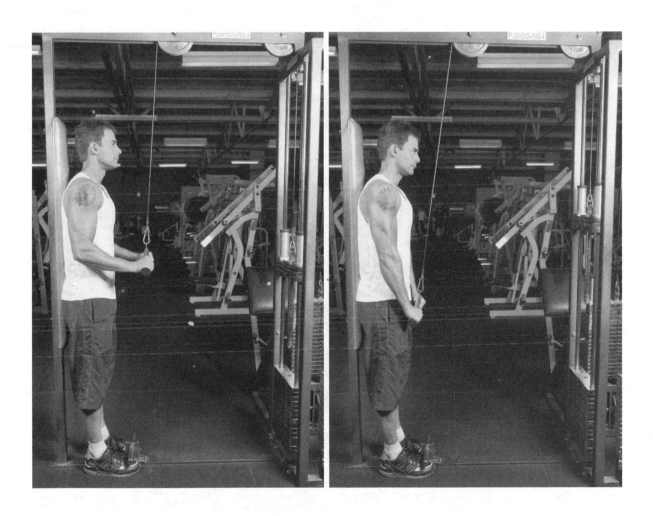

Lower Body (three sets of fifteen reps each)

SEATED LEG EXTENSIONS

Muscles worked: **Rectus femoris, vastus lateralis, vastus medialis, vastus intermedius (all quads)**

Sit down with your back against the padded support. Slide your lower legs beneath the padded lever, making sure that your knees are slightly beyond the edge of the seat to allow for comfortable extension. Extend legs until they are almost straight (do not allow knees to lock). Return to starting position. Repeat fifteen times.

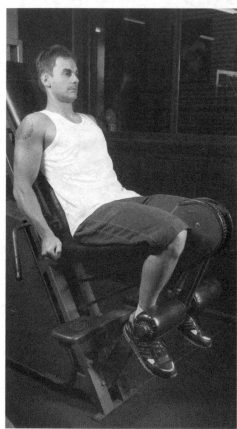
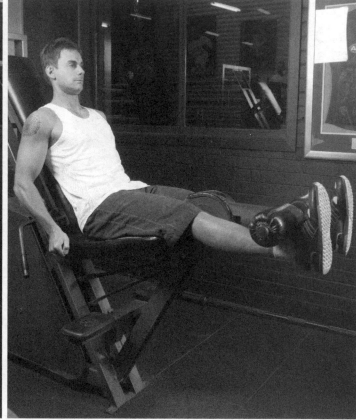

HAMSTRING CURLS

Major muscles worked: **Biceps femoris, semitendinosus, semimembranosus (hamstrings)**
Secondary muscles worked: **Gastrocnemius (calves)**

Lie face down on bench and lower your legs underneath the padded lever. Grasp handles beside the bench for stability. Slowly kick your legs back until the pad is almost touching your hamstrings. Return to starting position, being careful not to hyperextend your legs. Resist the urge to lift your upper body in an effort to gain momentum when kicking back. Repeat fifteen times.

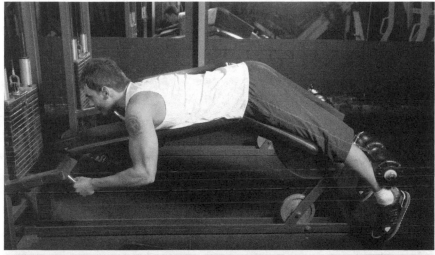

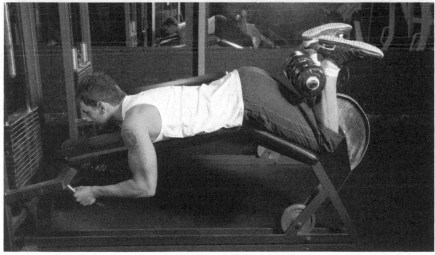

INCLINE HACK SQUAT MACHINE

Primary muscles worked: **Vastus medialis, vastus intermedius, vastus lateralis, rectus femoris (all quads)**

Secondary muscles worked: **Biceps femoris, semitendinosus, semimembranosus (all hamstrings), gluteus maximus (butt)**

Lean backward against padded back with your shoulders positioned under shoulder pads. Place your feet shoulder width apart in the center of the platform. Extend legs enough to release the side levers. Keep your abs tight and lower the weight down by bending knees until thighs are parallel to the platform. Return to standing (do not allow knees to lock). Repeat fifteen times.

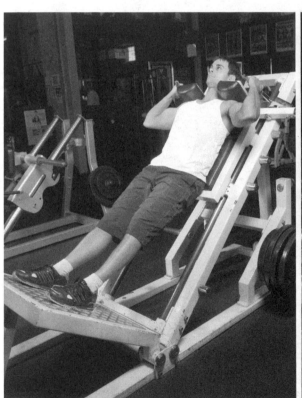
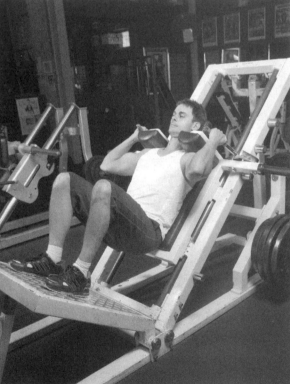

SEATED HAMSTRING CURLS

Muscles worked: **Biceps femoris, semimembranosus, semitendinosus, gastrocnemius (all hamstrings)**

Adjust the seat back so that when seated, your knees are over the edge of the seat and the stabilizing pad is across your upper shins. Hold the grips on the sides of the seat to keep your hips in place, and push your legs down, bending your knees to 90 degrees (no more). Hold for two seconds and slowly return to starting position (do not allow knees to lock). Repeat fifteen times.

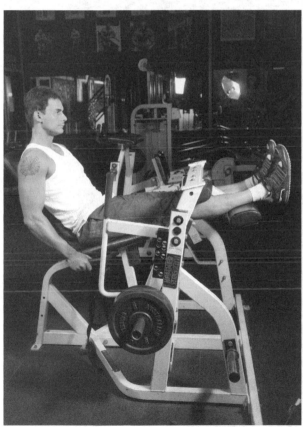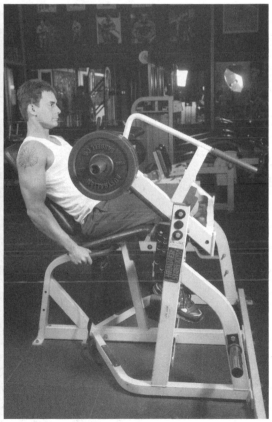

WALKING LUNGES WITH DUMBBELLS

Muscles worked: **Vastus medialis, vastus intermedius, vastus lateralis, rectus femoris (all quads), biceps femoris, semitendinosus, semimembranosus (hamstrings)**

Standing up straight with feet together, arms hanging down, palms facing in, and grasping a pair of dumbbells, take a slightly extended step forward with left leg. Lower both legs so that both knees are at a 90-degree angle, with your back knee almost touching the ground. Push up with front leg and bring back leg up and forward to starting position. Repeat action with right leg. Repeat ten times per side (for twenty total lunges).

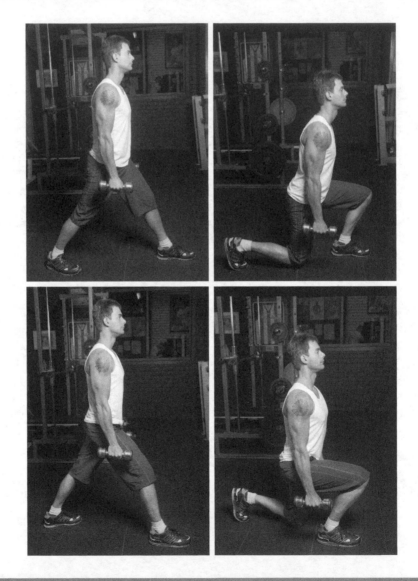

BARBELL STRAIGHT LEG DEAD LIFTS

Primary muscles worked: **Biceps femoris, semimembranosus, semitendinosus (all hamstrings)**
Secondary muscles worked: **Gluteus maximus (butt), adductor magnus (outer thigh),
erector spinae, trapezius (back), rhomboids (upper back)**

Standing with legs together and soft knees, grab barbell with an overhand grip and with hands on the outsides of the knees. Bend hips, keep back straight, and lower weight to the top of the feet. Keep barbell close to your shins as you lower the weight. Pause momentarily and then return to starting position. Repeat fifteen times.

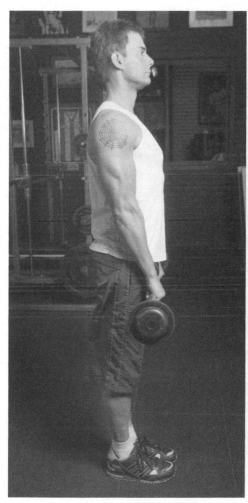
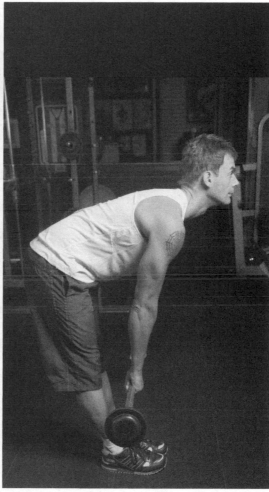

INCLINE LEG PRESS

Muscles worked: **Vastus medialis, vastus intermedius, vastus lateralis, rectus femoris (all quads), gluteus maximus, gluteus minimus (butt), biceps femoris, semimembranosus, semitendinosus (all hamstrings)**

Sit down on machine with your back against the back support. Place your feet hip width apart, feet flat, on the platform. Apply enough pressure to elevate the platform a few inches and release the side locks. Slowly lower platform, letting your knees bend in toward your chest, stopping before your lower back starts to lift off the back rest. Return to starting position (do not allow knees to lock). Repeat fifteen times. Don't forget to engage locks before resting.

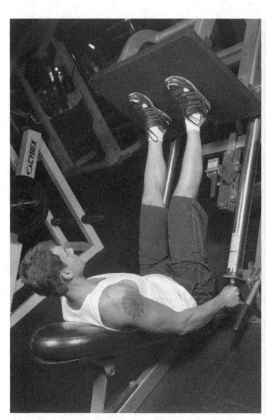
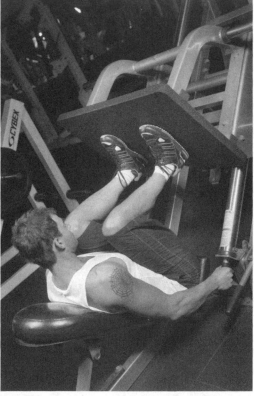

GLUTE KICKBACKS

Muscles worked: **Gluteus maximus (butt)**

Begin by getting on the floor on all fours with your knees behind your hips. Elevate your hips, keeping your back parallel with the ground. Rotate your left leg and push it toward the ceiling until the sole of your foot is parallel with the ceiling. Keep knee at the same angle throughout. Slowly lower to starting position, keeping the glutes tight. Repeat with right leg. Repeat ten times with each leg. (If using a glute machine, the angles are slightly different. Complete as depicted below.)

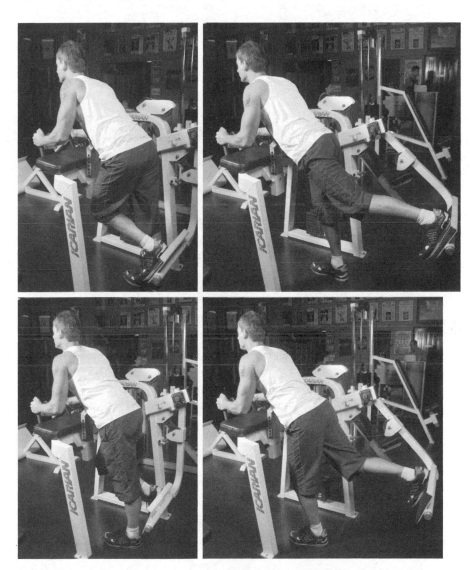

STANDING HAMSTRING CURLS

Muscles worked: **Biceps femoris, semimembranosus, semitendinosus (all hamstrings)**

Lean over machine with your chest against the padding. Place left leg in front of the roller. Place right knee on the padded support. With your left leg, slowly lift the roller, keeping the roller pressed against your Achilles tendon until the left knee is bent at about 90 degrees. Lower back to starting position. Repeat each leg fifteen times, for a total of thirty curls.

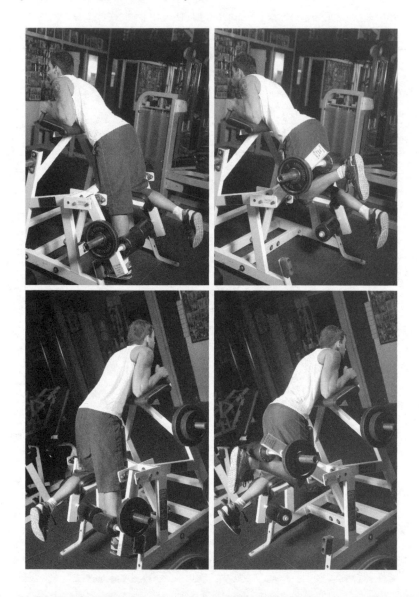

STANDING CALF RAISES

Primary muscles worked: **Gastrocnemius (calves)**
Secondary muscles worked: **Soleus (calves)**

Position shoulders under padding, with the balls of your feet on the platform and your arches and heels hanging off. Start in a squat position, push up against the pads until your body and legs are straight, and elevate heels, extending ankles as high as possible. Slowly lower down so your heels are slightly lower than the platform. Return to elevated position. Repeat fifteen times.

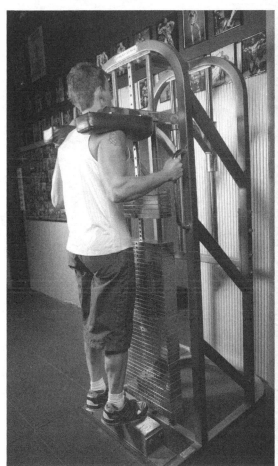 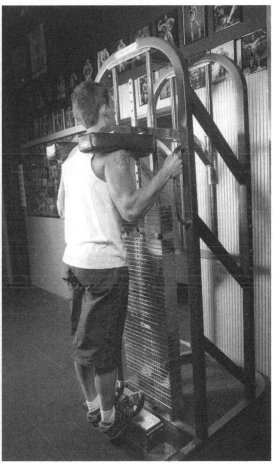

Ab Moves (Two sets of fifteen to twenty reps each)

Choose four of the following exercises per session:

AB CRUNCH (MACHINE)

Adjust the seat height to suit your frame and sit down with your back against the seat back. Anchor your legs against the ankle pads, tuck in your elbows, grab the handles, and pull them down so your chest moves toward your thighs as you crunch your torso. Keep your back pushed against the backrest at all times. Hold crunch position for two seconds and then return to starting position. Repeat twenty times.

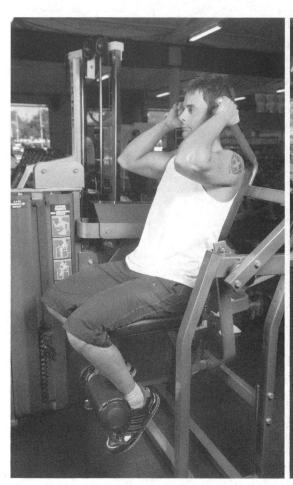 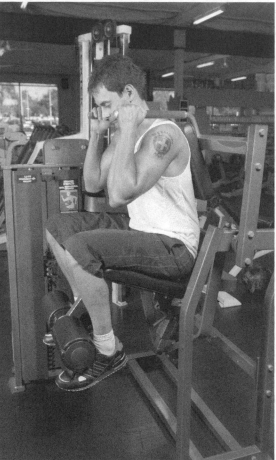

FLAT BENCH KNEE RAISES

Sit on the end of a flat bench, lean back slightly, and support your weight by holding onto the sides of the bench. Straighten your legs out away from the bench so they are almost parallel with the floor. Bend your knees and bring your thighs in toward your chest, keeping your abs contracted to relieve pressure on your back. Return to start position. Repeat twenty times.

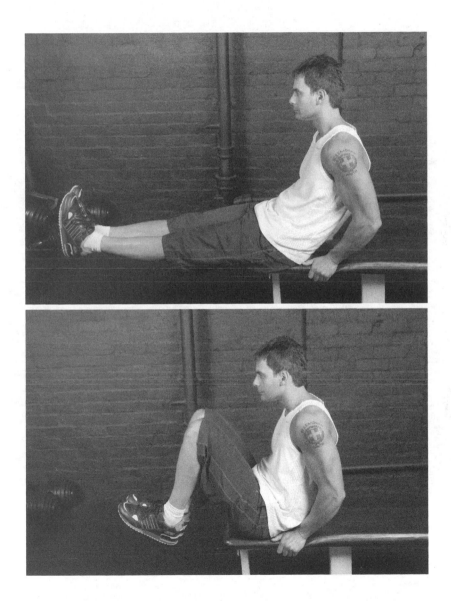

OBLIQUE CRUNCHES

Place a mat on the floor and lie on your back with your knees bent and feet flat on the floor. Drop your legs to one side. Keeping your lower back flat on the floor, place your hands behind your head and slowly lift both shoulders off the floor, using your abs, not your hands. Hold briefly. Return to start position. Repeat fifteen times on each side, for a total of thirty crunches.

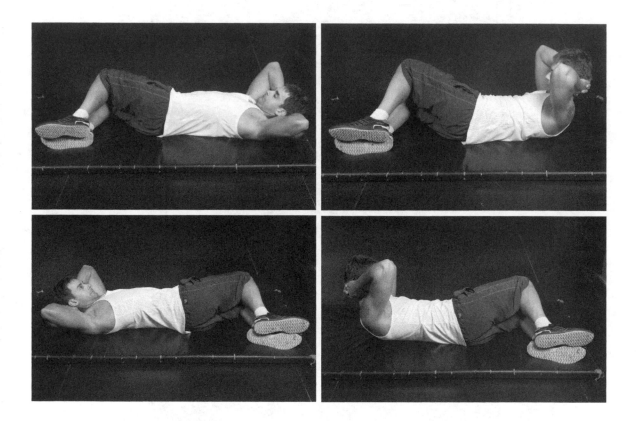

POLE TWISTS

Take a pole and rest it across your shoulder blades with your arms stretched out along the pole. Your legs should be a bit wider than shoulder width apart, your knees slightly bent and your toes pointing outward at a 45-degree angle. Lean forward slightly and twist your torso to one side until it is fully stretched. Return to middle, facing forward. Rotate your torso back to the other side until it is fully stretched. Keep your abs tight throughout the motion. Repeat twenty times on each side for a total of forty twists.

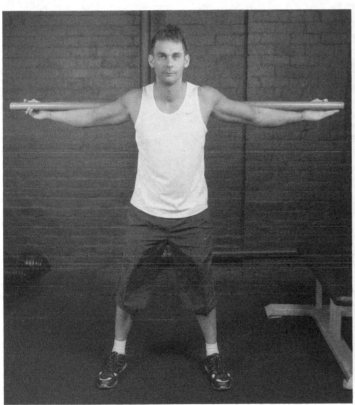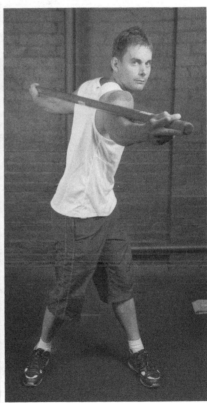

KEEP IT OFF

ROMAN CHAIR CRUNCHES

Position yourself in the Roman chair, with your elbows on support pads and lower back against the backrest. Bend your knees and raise your legs up until your thighs are parallel to the floor. (If that's too challenging, simply attempt to raise your knees up toward your chest—that will still help you burn calories and build strength. Even just hanging there with your knees bent is a success, but trust me, you will see progress quickly.) Squeeze abs and hold for two seconds. Slowly lower your legs back to starting position. Repeat twenty times.

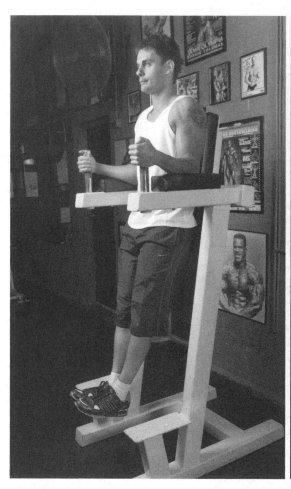 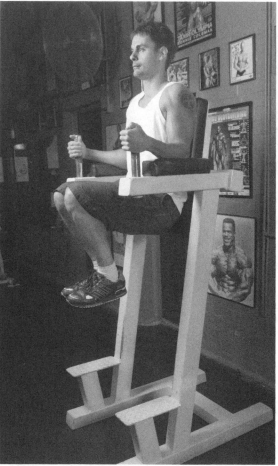

ADVANCED WORKOUT

This is the routine you will follow to shed the final 30 percent and reach your goal weight. The more complex exercises are ideal for toning one or two areas at a time.

The Advanced Workout bumps you up to five weekly weight sessions, none lasting more than fifty minutes. Rather than alternating between your upper and lower body, you'll cycle through different body parts. Men should complete three sets of eight to ten reps each (upper-body muscle groups) and three sets of ten to twelve reps each (lower body). Women should complete three sets of ten to twelve reps each for upper-body moves and three sets of twelve to fifteen reps each for the lower body. (Women will be using lighter weights, hence the increased repetitions.) Please note: this differs from the Beginner protocol. Strive for three days on, followed by a rest day, then another two days on, followed by one more rest day. Cardio will continue as before: Seven days a week, log fifteen minutes every morning on an empty stomach, supplemented by a brisk fifteen-minute post-dinner walk.

For best results, abdominal work should take place every second day and in the morning.

A typical week in the Advanced Workout will have you cycling through four weight workouts: Chest and triceps, back and biceps, shoulders and calves, quads and hamstrings. It will look like the chart on the following page.

Because there are only four different workouts but five weight-training sessions per week, one strength workout will be repeated every week. In other words, you won't always be working chest and triceps on Mondays or quads and hamstrings on Fridays; however, your rest days can remain the same.

Work Your Abs Without Even Trying

Free weights also work your core, which you'll use to stabilize your body as you complete your reps. So even when you think you're just working your shoulders or glutes, you're also strengthening your stomach and back.

PJ's
Pointer

	Monday	Tuesday	Wednesday	Thursday	Friday	Saturday	Sunday
7 a.m.	15 minutes of cardio Abs	15 minutes of cardio	15 minutes of cardio Abs	15 minutes of cardio	15 minutes of cardio Abs	15 minutes of cardio	15 minutes of cardio Abs
5 p.m.	Chest and triceps (Barbell Bench Press, Seated Pec Deck, Assisted Dips, Cable Crossovers, Dumbbell Pullovers on Flat Bench, Triceps Pushdowns, Overhead Rope Extensions, Dumbbell Triceps Kick-Backs)	Back and biceps (Assisted Pull-Ups, Lat Pulldowns, Seated Rows, Reverse Pec Deck, Cable Bicep Curls, Dumbbell Standing Bicep Curls, Seated Preacher Curls)	Shoulders and calves (Incline Shoulder Press, Seated Lateral Raises, Dumbbell Front Raises, Cable Lateral Raises, Dumbbell Shrugs, Standing Calf Raises, Calf Extensions on Incline Leg Press)	15-minute walk	Quads and hamstrings (Barbell Squats, Barbell Straight Leg Dead Lifts, Incline Hack Squat Machine, Hamstring Curls, Seated Leg Extensions, Seated Hamstring Curls, Walking Lunges with Dumbbells)	Chest and triceps (Barbell Bench Press, Seated Pec Deck, Assisted Dips, Cable Crossovers, Dumbbell Pullovers on Flat Bench, Triceps Pushdowns, Overhead Rope Extensions, Dumbbell Triceps Kick-Backs)	15-minute walk
Evening	15-minute walk	15-minute walk	15-minute walk	15-minute walk	15-minute walk	15-minute walk	15-minute walk

Monday: morning cardio and abs, evening chest and triceps, evening cardio
Tuesday: morning cardio, evening back and biceps, evening cardio
Wednesday: morning cardio and abs, evening shoulders and calves, evening cardio
Thursday: morning and evening cardio, no weights or abs
Friday: morning cardio and abs, evening quads and hamstrings, evening cardio
Saturday: morning cardio, evening chest and triceps, evening cardio
Sunday: morning and evening cardio and abs, no weights

Chest and Triceps

BARBELL BENCH PRESS

Lie down on the bench and grasp bar with your hands overhead and a wide grip. Push up slightly to dismount barbell and lower weight to your chest. Press upward until arms are fully extended (do not allow elbows to lock). Repeat ten times.

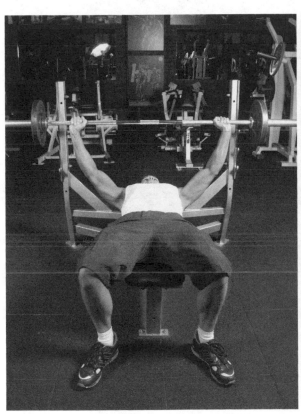 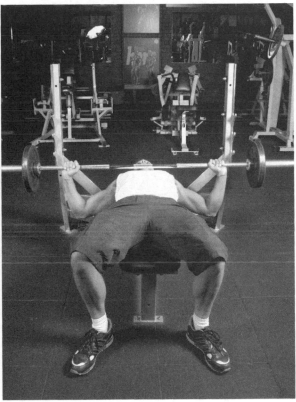

SEATED PEC DECK

Sit down with back facing the pad. Reaching back one at a time, grip handles on either side. Squeeze your clenched fists together so that they nearly touch (but don't actually touch) in front of you. Slowly return to the starting position. Repeat ten times.

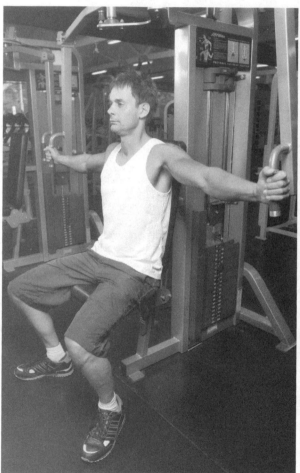 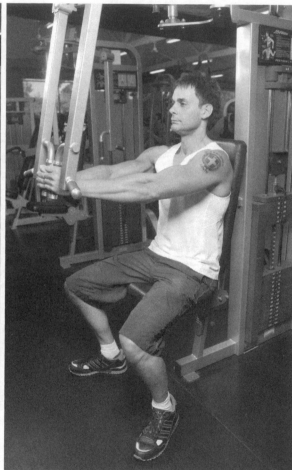

ASSISTED DIPS

On a weighted dips machine choose the desired weight level (weight is used to counterbalance body weight). Facing the machine, grasp handles with an overhand grip and kneel on the padded platform. Keeping your back straight and upright, bend your elbows and lower your body down until your upper arms are parallel to the floor. Return to starting position. Repeat ten times.

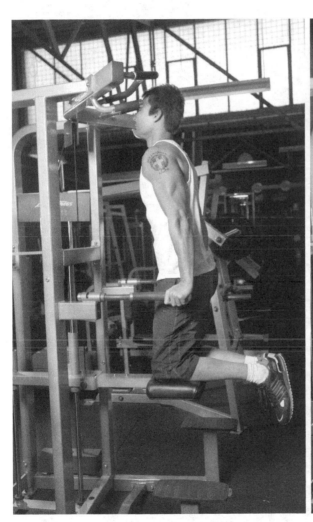
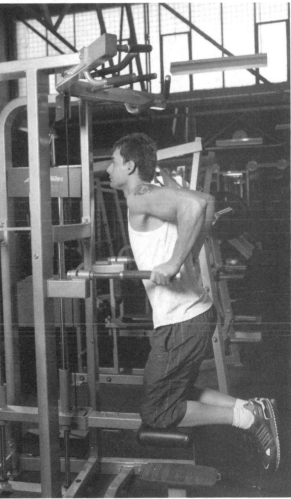

CABLE CROSSOVERS

Stand in the center of a cable pulley machine with your feet apart for stability. Grab a handle in each hand with an overhand grip so you form a "T" position. Put one foot slightly forward and lean forward, keeping your back straight. Draw handles down with your arms slightly bent at the elbows, bringing cables together in front of you with your palms facing inward. Hold for two seconds and return to starting position. Repeat ten times.

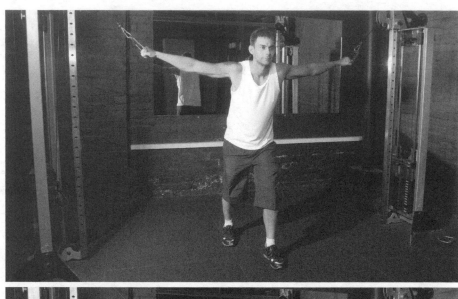

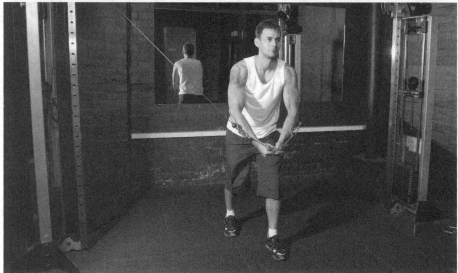

DUMBBELL PULLOVERS ON FLAT BENCH

Holding one dumbbell with both hands under inner plate of dumbbell, lay down on a bench with your head slightly over the end of the bench, feet flat on the floor, and arms extended toward the ceiling. While maintaining a slight bend in your elbows, lower your arms out in a wide arc toward the floor until your hands are in line with your shoulders. Return to starting position. Repeat ten times.

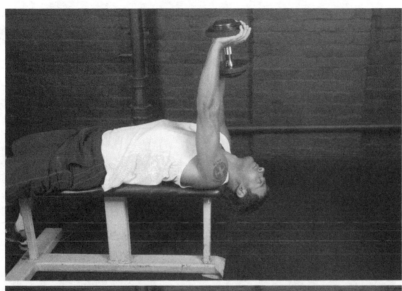

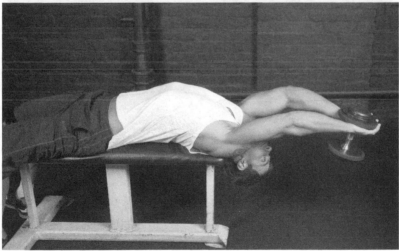

TRICEPS PUSHDOWNS

Stand facing a high pulley with a straight bar or V bar. Grip the bar, palms down, a bit narrower than shoulder width and bring the bar down so your elbows are close to your body, and your forearms, when parallel to the floor, are waist level. Continue pushing down until arms are nearly extended. Pause for two seconds and then return forearms to waist level. Repeat ten times.

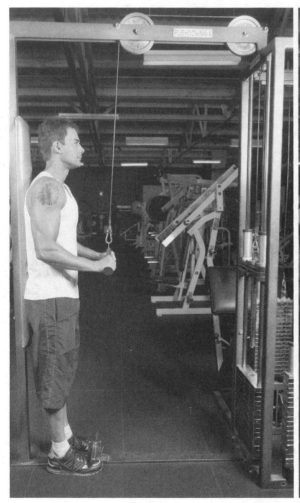
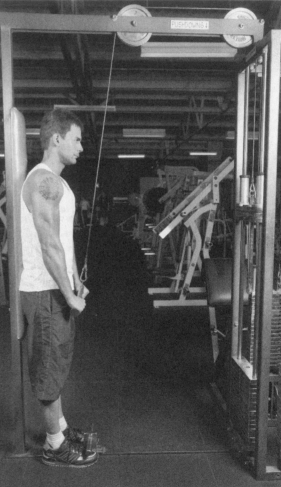

OVERHEAD ROPE EXTENSIONS

Stand with your back to a high pulley and reach overhead with the rope in your hand. Take one step forward to elevate the weight stack. Keeping your back straight and hips slightly forward, with your thumbs above your head and elbows facing straight ahead, extend your arms until they are fully extended and twist the rope so that your palms face the ground. Slowly allow arms to bend back to starting position. Repeat ten times.

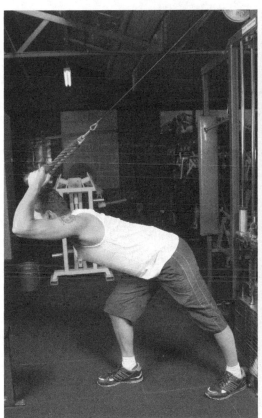
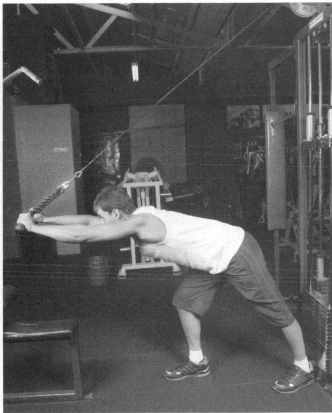

DUMBBELL TRICEPS KICKBACKS

Grasping a dumbbell in your left hand, bend over and kneel your right leg onto a bench, supporting yourself with your right arm. Keeping your upper left arm parallel to the floor, extend your forearm until it is almost straight (do not lock your elbow). Return and repeat ten times. Switch sides and repeat.

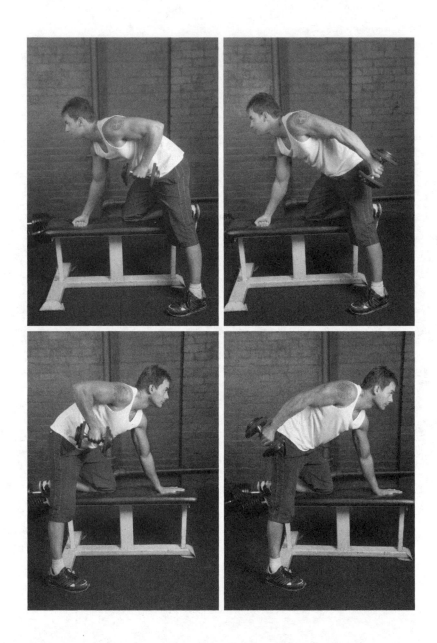

ASSISTED PULL-UPS

On a weighted pull-ups machine, choose the desired weight level (weight is used to counterbalance body weight). Facing the machine, kneel on the padded platform and reach up to hold the handles with your wrists facing forward. Keep your back straight and lower your body down until your arms are straight (do not allow your elbows to lock). Return to starting position, squeezing through your upper back. Repeat ten times.

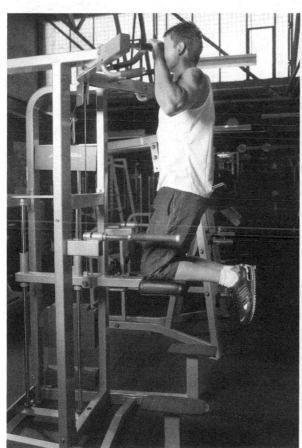
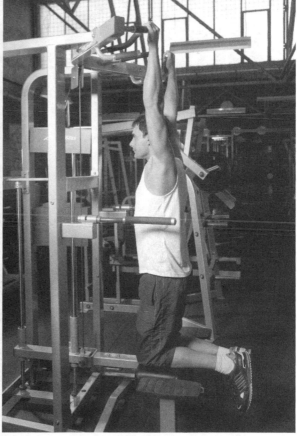

LAT PULLDOWNS

Grasp the bar with a wide grip and slowly sit down, sliding your knees underneath the pads. Pull the bar down smoothly until it touches the top of your chest, being careful not to hike your shoulders up beforehand. Extend your arms back up. Repeat ten times.

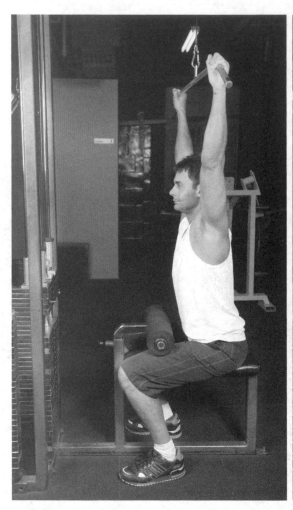
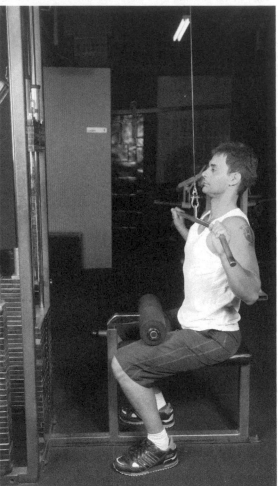

SEATED ROWS

Sit on the bench with knees slightly bent, feet slightly parted, back straight, and cable handles in hand (palms facing in). Pulling your shoulder blades back and down and contracting your core, pull your elbows back until they are at your sides and push your chest out. Return to starting position in a controlled manner, being careful not to let your shoulders slump forward or ride up. Repeat ten times.

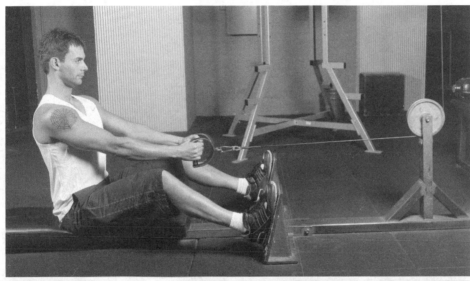

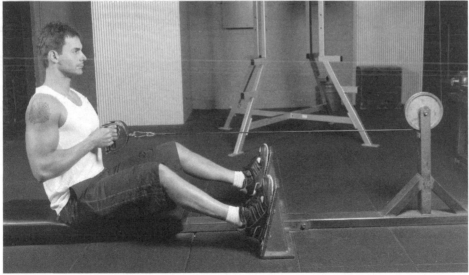

REVERSE PEC DECK

Sit facing a pec deck machine, resting your chest against the padded back and keeping your torso as straight as possible. Grab the handles and slightly bend arms at the elbow. In a controlled fashion push your arms out and back as far as possible. Keep your core engaged the whole time. Slowly return to start. Repeat ten times.

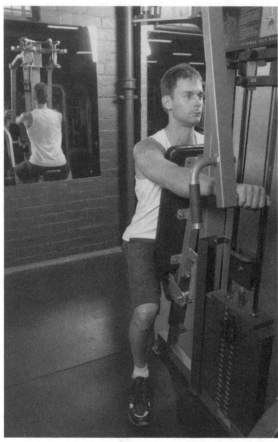
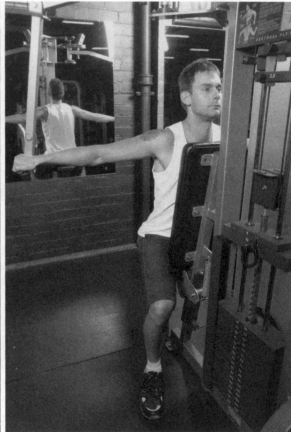

CABLE BICEP CURLS

Standing close to the machine with knees slightly bent, grasp a low pulley cable bar with your hands shoulder width apart and your palms facing up. Curl the bar up until your forearms touch your biceps, making sure to keep your elbows tucked in. Lower back to starting position. Repeat ten times.

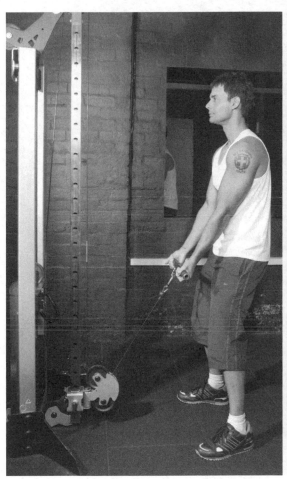 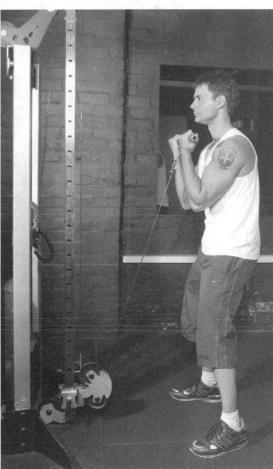

DUMBBELL STANDING BICEP CURLS

Begin by standing with feet hip width apart, holding a dumbbell in each hand with your arms hanging straight down and your palms facing forward. Keeping your elbows tucked in, raise and curl one side, raising your forearm until it touches your bicep and your palm faces your shoulder. Lower to starting position and repeat with opposite arm. Repeat ten times.

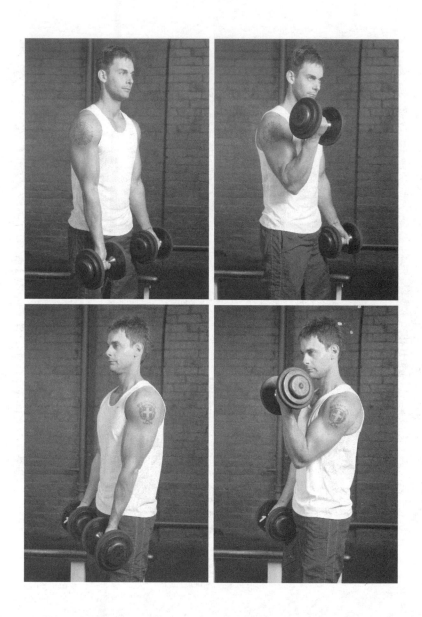

SEATED PREACHER CURLS

Sit down on a preacher bench and rest your upper arms on the pad. Grasp the curl bar with your hands shoulder width apart and an underhand grip. Curl the bar until your forearms touch your biceps. Lower back to starting position. Repeat ten times.

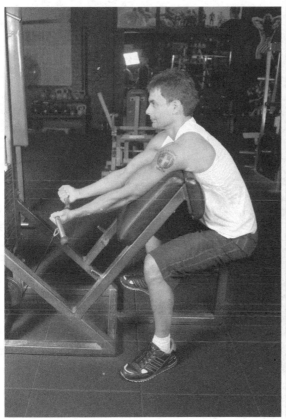
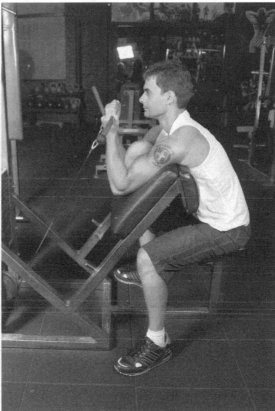

Shoulders and Calves

INCLINE SHOULDER PRESS

Sitting down, grasp the handles with an overhand grip. Push upward until your arms are fully extended overhead (do not lock your elbows). Lower back to starting position. Repeat ten times.

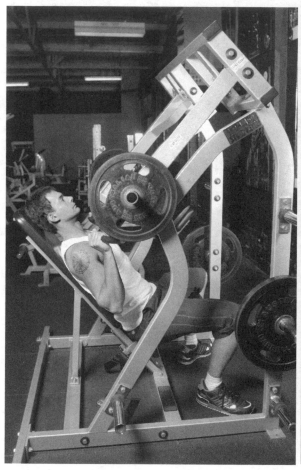

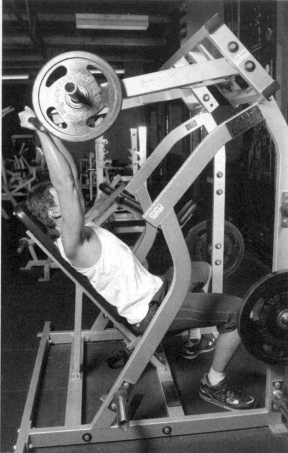

SEATED LATERAL RAISES

Sitting on a bench with a vertical backrest, grasp a dumbbell in each hand (choose the lightest weight first to test), with your palms facing in, arms hanging down, and elbows slightly bent. Raise both arms up and out to the sides until they are parallel with the floor. Slowly return to starting position. Repeat ten times.

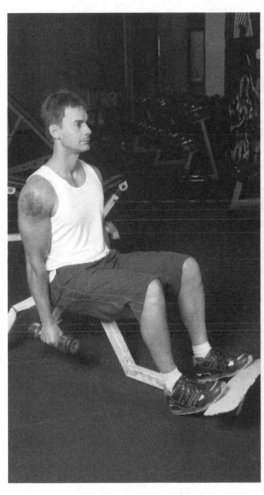
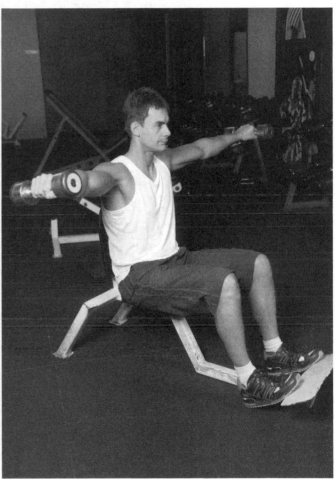

DUMBBELL FRONT RAISES

Standing with feet hip width apart, grasp a dumbbell in each hand (choose the lightest weight first to test), with your palms facing down, slightly in front of your upper legs and your elbows slightly bent. One at a time, raise your arm up and out in front of you until it is parallel with the floor. Slowly return to starting position. Repeat ten times per side, for a total of twenty raises.

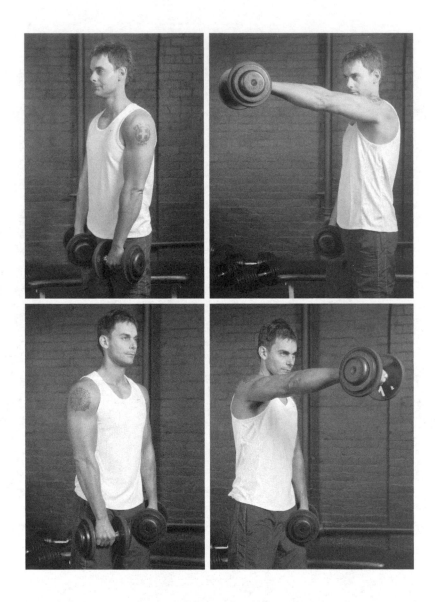

CABLE LATERAL RAISES

Stand to one side of the cable crossover machine with soft knees and a contracted core. Making sure the handles of the pulleys are in the lowermost position, grasp handle with your opposite hand, your palm facing the pulley, and your opposite shoulder leaning toward the weight stack. With your elbow slightly bent, pull the handle back across your body, straighten your torso, and extend your arm until it is parallel to the floor. Hold for two seconds and slowly return to start position. Repeat ten times on each side, for a total of twenty raises.

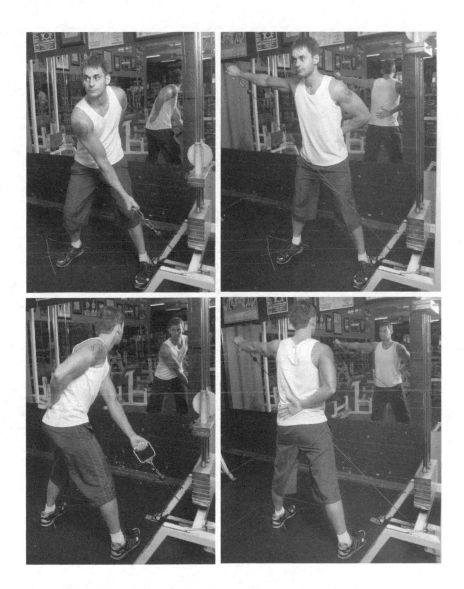

DUMBBELL SHRUGS

In a standing position and holding a dumbbell in each hand (choose the lightest weight first to test), hang your arms down and face your palms in. Shrug your shoulders as high as possible and hold for two seconds. Lower back to starting position. Repeat ten times.

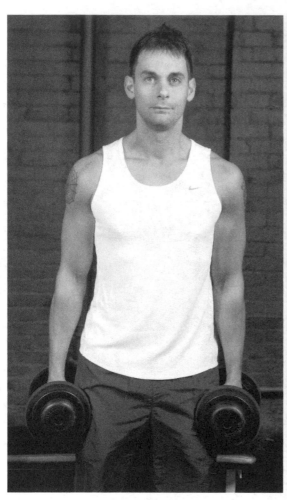
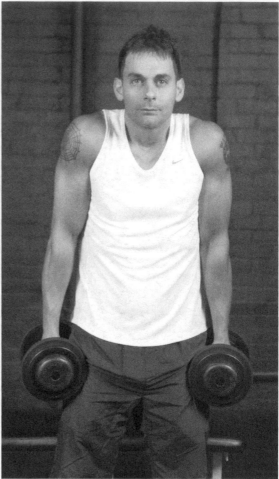

STANDING CALF RAISES

Position your shoulders under padding, with the balls of your feet on the platform and your arches and heels hanging off. Start in a squat position; push up against the pads until your body and legs are straight. Elevate your heels, extending your ankles as high as possible. Slowly lower down so your heels are slightly lower than the platform. Return to elevated position. Repeat twelve times.

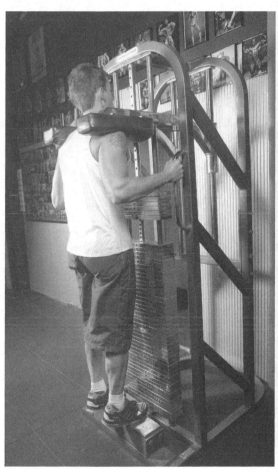 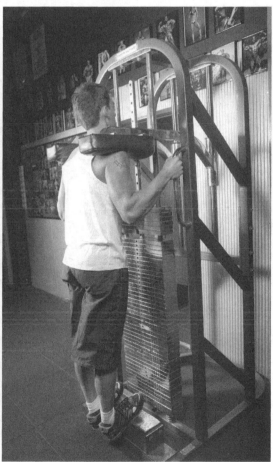

CALF EXTENSIONS ON INCLINE LEG PRESS

Sit down on incline leg press machine, with your back against the back support. Place your feet slightly wider than hip width apart on the platform, with your toes and the balls of your feet on the platform and heels and arches off the bottom edge of the platform. Push the platform with your toes until your knees are locked and your legs are straight, then fully extend ankles and hold for two seconds. Bend your ankles back the other way until your calves are fully stretched. Repeat twelve times. (Keep side locks engaged at all times to prevent the platform from falling and causing serious injury.)

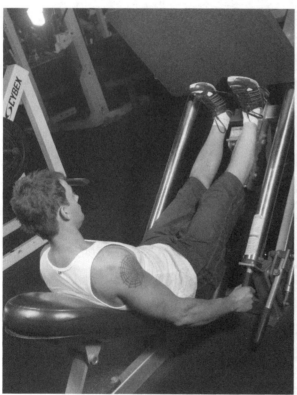 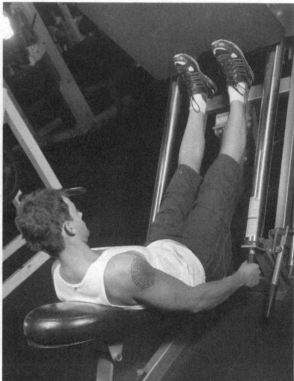

BARBELL SQUATS

Complete your first set with a light weight as a warm up, your feet shoulder width apart. Position the bar high on the back of your shoulders and grip it, with a wide, overhand grip rotated to a "shot put" position. Keeping your back straight, push your hips back and bend your knees to lower your body down as if you are about to sit, until your thighs are parallel to the floor. Return to starting position until your legs are straight. Repeat twelve times.

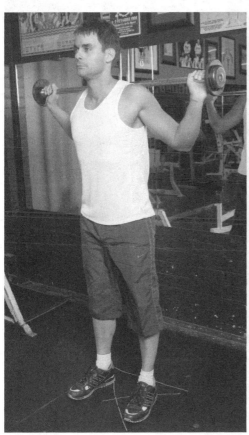
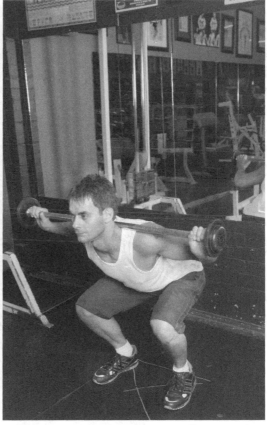

BARBELL STRAIGHT LEG DEAD LIFTS

Standing with your legs together and soft knees, grab a barbell with an overhand grip and your hands on the outsides of your knees. Bend your hips, keeping your back straight, and lower the weight to the top of your feet. Keep the barbell close to your shins as you lower the weight. Pause momentarily and then return to starting position. Repeat twelve times.

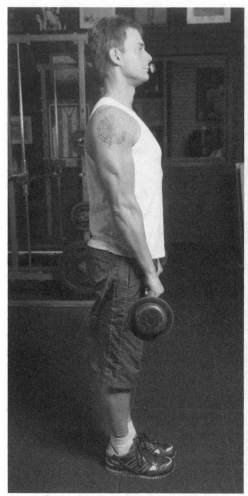
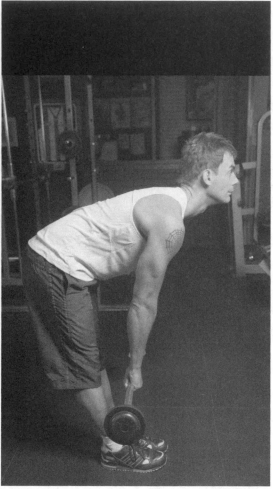

INCLINE HACK SQUAT MACHINE

Lean backward against the padded back with your shoulders positioned under the shoulder pads. Place your feet shoulder width apart in the center of the platform. Extend your legs enough to release the side levers. Keep your abs tight, and lower the weight down by bending your knees until your thighs are parallel to the platform. Return to standing (do not allow your knees to lock). Repeat twelve times.

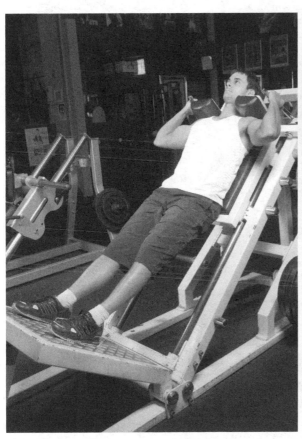
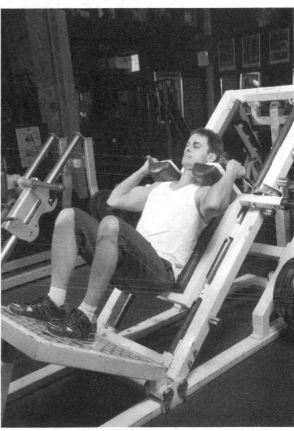

HAMSTRING CURLS

Lie face-down on bench, lowering legs underneath the padded lever. Grasp the handles beside the bench for stability. Slowly kick your legs back until the pad is almost touching your hamstrings. Return to starting position, being careful not to hyperextend your legs. Resist the urge to lift your upper body in an effort to gain momentum when kicking back. Repeat twelve times.

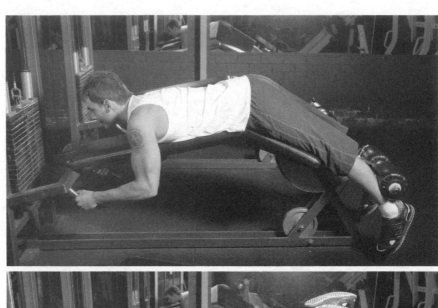

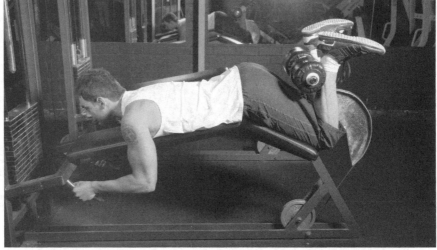

SEATED LEG EXTENSIONS

Sit down with your back against the padded support. Slide your lower legs beneath the padded lever, making sure that your knees are slightly beyond the edge of the seat so as to allow for comfortable extension. Extend your legs until they are almost straight (do not allow your knees to lock). Return to starting position. Repeat twelve times.

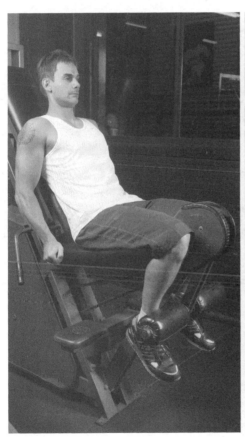
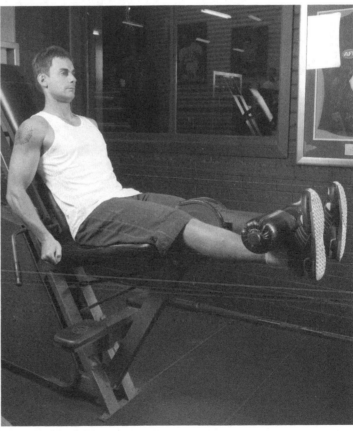

KEEP IT OFF

SEATED HAMSTRING CURLS

Adjust the seat back so that, when seated, your knees are over the edge of the seat and the stabilizing pad is across your thighs. Hold the grips on the sides of the seat to keep your hips in place, and push your legs down, bending your knees to 90 degrees (no more). Hold for two seconds and then slowly return to starting position (do not allow knees to lock). Repeat fifteen times.

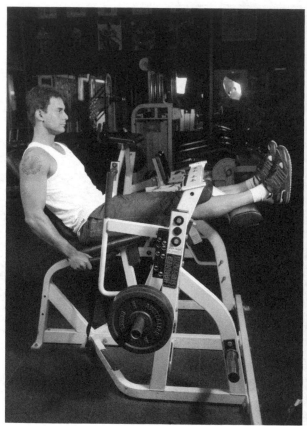
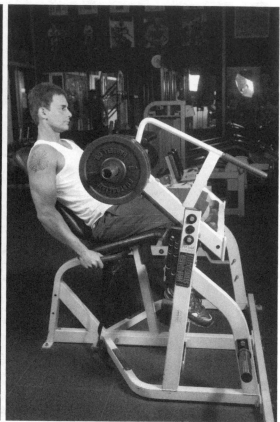

WALKING LUNGES WITH DUMBBELLS

Standing up straight with your feet together, arms hanging down, palms facing in, and grasping a pair of dumbbells, take a slightly extended step forward with left leg. Lower both your legs so that both knees are at a 90-degree angle, with your back knee almost touching the ground. Push up with your front leg and bring your back leg up and forward to starting position. Repeat this action with your right leg. Repeat ten times per side, for a total of twenty lunges.

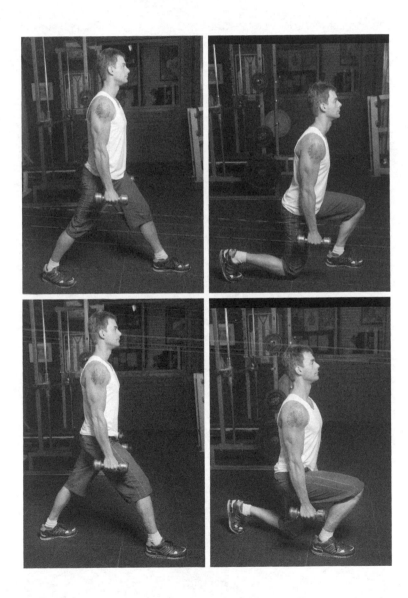

KEEP IT OFF

Stretching

Between each set of exercises take time to stretch the corresponding muscles. These moves can be done quickly, right next to the machine you are working on, to maximize time efficiency. Hold each stretch for five to ten seconds.

CHEST

Reach both hands behind your back and intertwine your fingers. Gently reach hands away from your body until you feel a stretch across the chest.

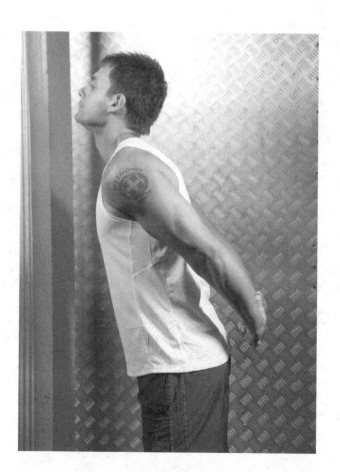

CHEST

Place your right hand on a doorjamb or tall, sturdy machine at chest level. Rotate your body to the left until you feel a stretch in your right chest and armpit. Repeat on your left side.

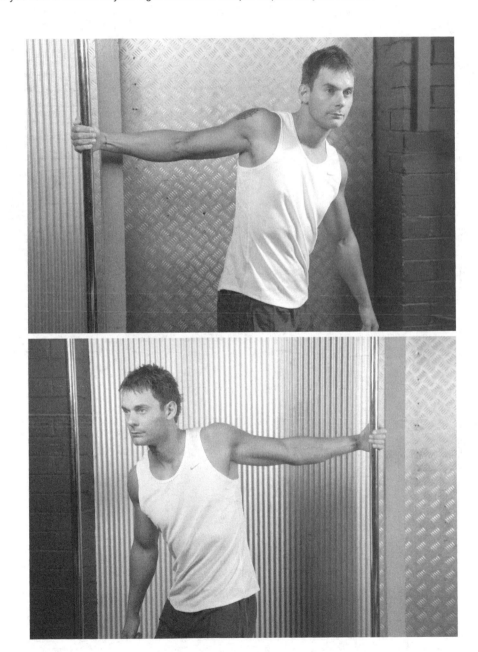

BACK

Face a piece of sturdy equipment and take a small step to the right. Squatting down, grab the equipment with your right hand (your right arm should cross slightly in front of you) and lean slightly to the right until you feel a stretch in the right side of your back and arm. Repeat on your left side.

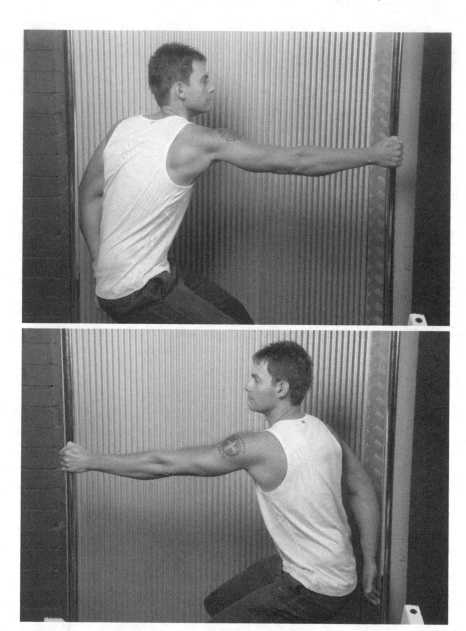

BACK

Standing with your knees soft (not locked), place your hands on your lower back and gently bend backward.

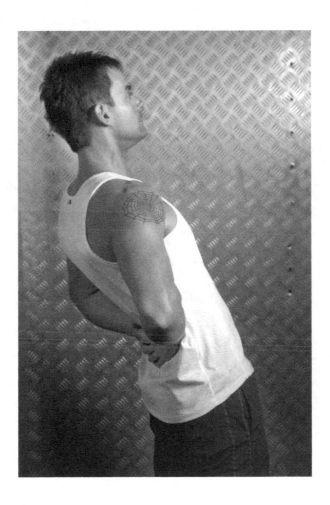

SHOULDERS

Reach your right arm across your body at chest level and use your left arm to hug your right arm close to your chest until you feel a stretch in your right shoulder. Repeat on your left side.

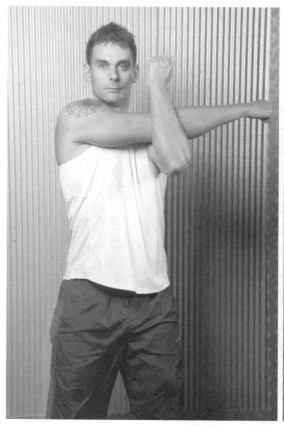
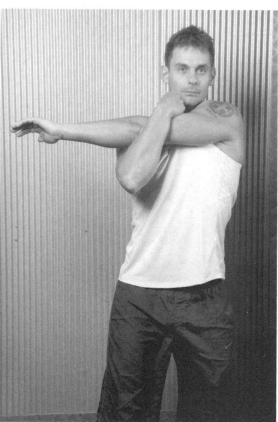

SHOULDERS

Face a piece of sturdy equipment or pole and bend over from your waist and grasp equipment at chest level. Pull your body away from the pole to stretch through your shoulders.

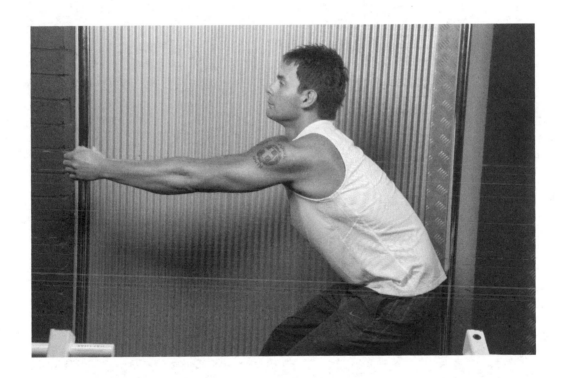

BICEPS

Extend your right arm out in front of your body and rotate it so your palm is facing up. Use your left hand to gently pull down on your right fingertips until you feel a stretch in your right biceps. Repeat on your left side.

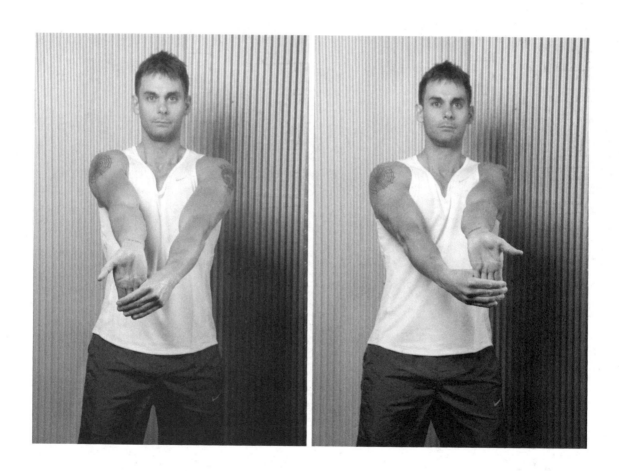

TRICEPS

Raise your right arm overhead and bend at your elbow, so your right hand is reaching behind your head and toward the middle of your back. Use your left arm to push down gently on your right arm until you feel a stretch in your right triceps. Repeat on your left side.

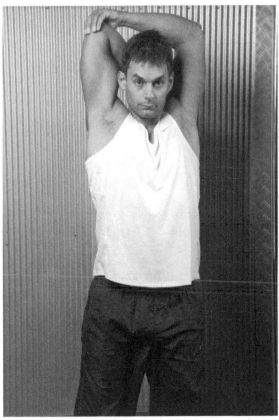 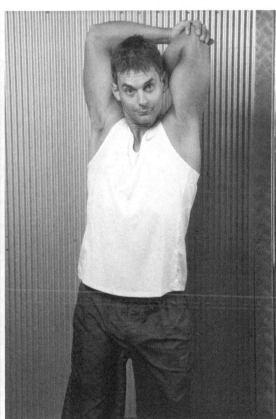

QUADRICEPS

Standing with soft knees, bend your right leg at the knee. Reach back with your right hand to grab your right ankle. Keeping both knees together, gently push your hips forward until you feel a stretch in your right quad. Repeat on your left side. You may use a pole for stability.

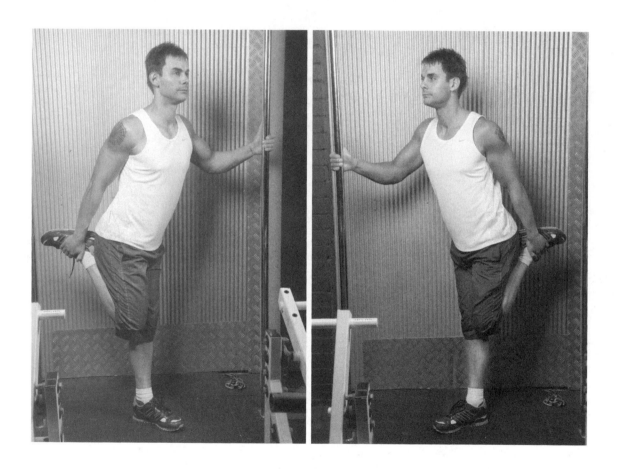

QUADRICEPS

Step forward with your right foot into a wide lunge. Not allowing your right knee to extend past your toes, drop down until you feel a stretch in your left quad. Repeat on your left side. You may use a pole for stability.

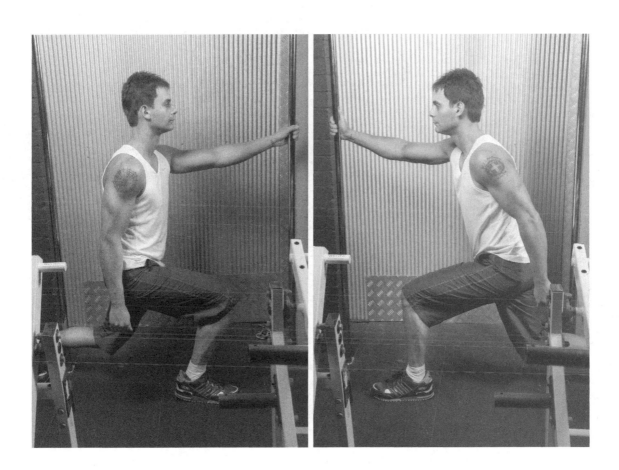

KEEP IT OFF

HAMSTRINGS

Place your right foot on a sturdy surface, about mid-thigh height. Keeping your leg straight and locked, bend forward from your waist and reach toward your ankle until you feel a stretch in your right hamstring. Repeat on your left side.

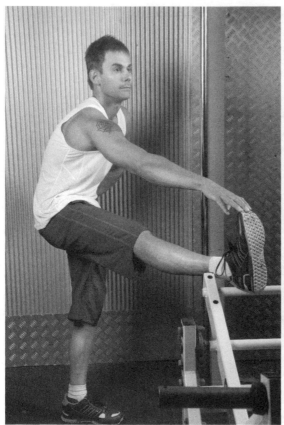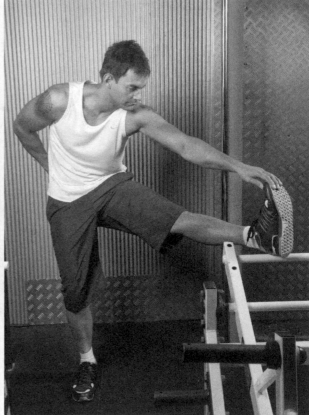

HAMSTRINGS

Standing with your feet together and legs straight and locked, bend forward from your waist and reach for your toes until you feel a stretch in your hamstrings. Keep your back as straight as possible.

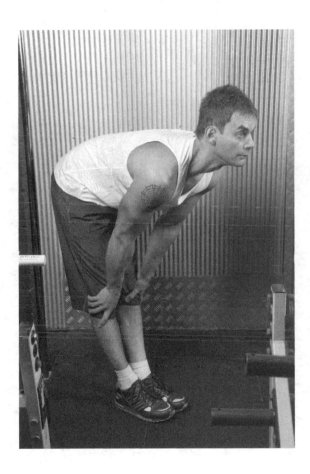

CALVES

Standing about four feet away from a wall or pole, plant your left foot in front of your right and reach for the wall. Keeping both heels on the floor, lean into the wall until you feel a stretch in your right calf. After holding for five to ten seconds, bend your back (right) leg and hold the stretch. Repeat on your left side.

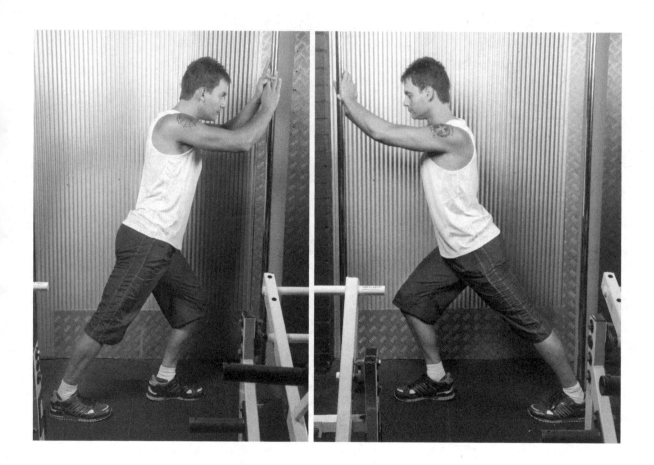

ABDOMINALS

Lie facedown on a mat. Place your hands on the floor and in front of your shoulders. Push your upper body off the floor and arch your back until you feel a stretch in your abdominals. Do not lock out your arms or let your shoulders shrug up. Keep your shoulder blades tucked in.

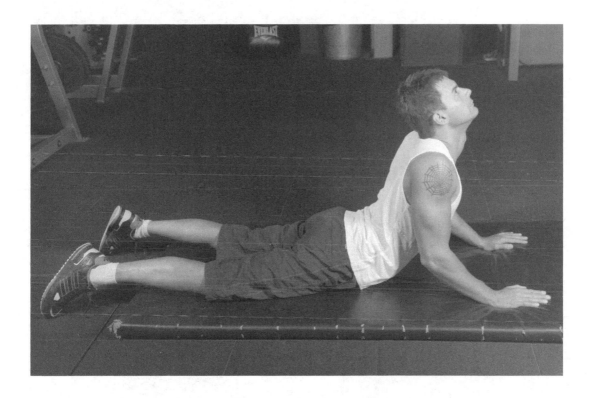

OBLIQUES

Standing with your feet shoulder width apart, slide your left arm down the side of your left leg as your reach your right arm overhead and to the left. Keep your right shoulder back. Keep reaching until you feel a stretch in your right side. Repeat on your left side.

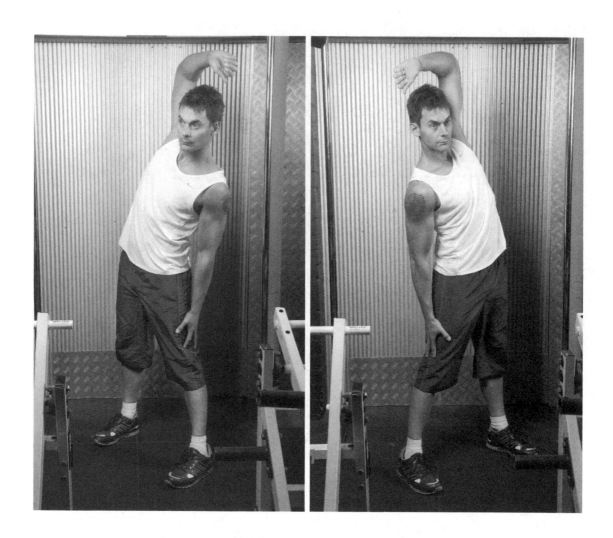

THE NIGHTTIME WALK

The evening walk burns more calories and promotes a good night's sleep. If you eat dinner and go straight to bed, your body, in a sense, stays awake, working throughout the night to metabolize your meal. The result: restless slumber and major brain fog the next day. Allowing your evening meal to settle for forty-five minutes and taking a brisk walk will stimulate your metabolism, helping it to process dinner. Stick to fifteen minutes—twenty, max—at a continuous brisk pace, and follow it up with a cup of herbal tea to detoxify and calm your body down even more. A hot shower will relax you even further, priming you for a peaceful sleep. You'll wake up refreshed and ready for your morning cardio. These evening walks will give you that extra edge, delivering even quicker results.

THE MAINTENANCE PHASE

Essentially, the Advanced Workout *is* the Maintenance Workout. This is the routine I myself still follow to this day. Once you've reached your goal weight, you'll have become familiar with the moves, you'll know the layout of your gym like the back of your hand, and you'll feel in total control of your workout. If you want to change things up, try incorporating different forms of cardio, like Spin class, hiking, Zumba, or another group-aerobics class. You'll be stronger and will have greater endurance and cardio capacity, so you can absolutely tackle activities that are more challenging than a fast walk or the Elliptical machine. (That said, my personal cardio equipment of choice remains, to this

Entrepreneurs, Take Note! **PJ's** Pointer

I know it sounds strange, but I find that clients who work nine-to-five–type jobs in offices tend to do quite well at weight loss, whereas business owners and entrepreneurs are sometimes less open to following someone else's protocol. Those are the clients who tend to make little changes here and there, like skipping a certain move or doing thirty minutes of cardio instead of fifteen, thinking they know best. Here's what I tell them: you own your own law practice because you're an excellent lawyer. But fitness is what I excel in. I know my business just as well as you know yours. Follow my lead and I'll help you succeed.

day, the Elliptical cross-trainer. I just love how it torches fat while remaining non-impact, so it's easy on the joints.)

At this point you'll likely find that you can spend less time in the gym while maintaining the same results. But if you start backsliding and see changes in your body that you don't like, that means it's time to step things back up. Pull out KO-90 and start following the Advanced Workout to the letter. Your muscles will remember the moves, and you'll be back on track in no time.

It boils down to this: with KO-90 you'll make some sacrifices in order to reach your end goal in a safe, efficient manner. Then it's time to live by your own rules, which will no longer include hours spent on the couch, watching TV, or consuming monstrous portions of high sugar, fatty foods, and dairy. You'll have a stellar new body, a renewed sense of confidence, and energy to burn. I promise I will deliver you to a place where you *will* achieve your goals and enjoy the kind of healthy, satisfied life you've always dreamed of. Then, it'll be up to you to start living on your own terms. And I promise you—it will feel awesome.

Ninety days. Three months. It's really not all that long, especially considering what you'll be giving yourself in return. A lifetime of Strength. Endurance. Health. Self-esteem. You'll stand taller, knowing you're living your best life, Let KO-90 take—and keep—you there.

PART 6

GET MOTIVATED

The Secrets of Their—and Your—Success

You've been hearing from some of my clients throughout the book; now here's your chance to meet them and hear more about their amazing successes using KO-90.

DORA DOGAS, age thirty-five

STARTING WEIGHT: 374 pounds
CURRENT WEIGHT: 176 pounds
POUNDS LOST: 198
POUNDS AWAY FROM GOAL WEIGHT: 20

Why I wanted to lose weight: I suffered from high blood pressure, back pain, swollen feet, iron deficiency, and obstructive sleep apnea that was so severe I needed an oxygen mask to sleep. Despite having gastric bypass surgery, I continued to gain weight as I turned to food for emotional comfort. Seatbelts couldn't reach around my body, and I didn't fit into my bathtub. I was sick of strangers staring at me, which made me feel worthless. I hated looking in the mirror, and wanted a happier life for myself.

My biggest obstacle: I had tried diets, gyms, women's only gyms, meal delivery, shakes, meal replacements, other trainers, and gastric banding in an attempt to limit the food I ate. I took a taxi to the gym—just two blocks from my home. I didn't *believe* I could lose weight. But PJ was not deterred. His strong belief in his clients' capacity to achieve their goal makes all the difference. PJ gave me the tools to shrink from a size 30 to a size 6 and have my gastric band removed.

PJ's best advice: To keep on trying and believe in my ability to achieve my goals.

ANDREW FEDOROWICZ, age sixty-two

STARTING WEIGHT: 284 pounds
CURRENT WEIGHT: 236 pounds
POUNDS LOST: 48
POUNDS AWAY FROM GOAL WEIGHT: 16

Why I wanted to lose weight: I needed to feel better and lower my risk of diabetes. My wife, Amanda, whom I love to bits, said to me on more than one occasion, "Do something about it while you are still capable of making a choice."

My biggest obstacle: I love good food and good wine, and I'm married to the world's best cook. Having to succumb to a comparatively understated food program was very difficult at first. But despite a rocky start, I quickly began to enjoy eating clean. I was sad to pour my Paul Newman Caesar Salad Dressing down the drain, but now I enjoy my vegetables with balsamic vinegar. I look forward to my tuna salad "prelunch" at 11.30 a.m. every day. My doctor cannot believe my results—I used to be borderline diabetic and had a blood pressure of 160/95. Now it's 120/60. I feel like I'm going to be the first human being to live to 130! PJ has given me back my life. The only downside is I need a whole new wardrobe. My belts now have five to eight spare holes, and everything just hangs off me. It's a great problem to have.

PJ's best advice: I will never forget when he told me, "Commit yourself to me for three months and I will change your life, forever." And he has.

> **STARTING WEIGHT:** 168 pounds
> **CURRENT WEIGHT:** 135 pounds
> **POUNDS LOST:** 33
> **POUNDS AWAY FROM GOAL WEIGHT:** 8

Why I wanted to lose weight: Seven years ago I weighed 132 pounds and worked out hard to maintain it. Then I got married and let myself go. My husband is a fitness freak, and he has motivated me to get back into a routine.

My biggest obstacle: Time. Running your own business doesn't allow you the flexibility or time to truly commit to a plan—or so I thought, until I met PJ. Also, for many years I was so crazed with work that I would only eat once a day, late at night after working a sixteen-hour day. I have been able to overcome all of this since starting my journey with PJ's help. He showed me how to plan my schedule so I can make time for everything—work, fitness, food, and family.

PJ's best advice: When it comes to cardio, less is more.

BERNADETTE CLAREBROUGH, age fifty-one

STARTING WEIGHT: 194 pounds
CURRENT WEIGHT: 141 pounds
POUNDS LOST: 53
POUNDS AWAY FROM GOAL WEIGHT: 0—reached her goal!

Why I wanted to lose weight: From the ages of twenty-two to twenty-nine I tried several rapid weight-loss methods, including diet pills (basically uppers), diuretics, growth-hormone injections, extreme low-calorie food plans, laxatives, and excessive exercise. I did drop weight and was, at times, quite skinny, but it was nearly impossible to maintain, and this led to bingeing. At twenty-nine my extreme dieting methods led to a stroke.

Basically, I woke up one day and realized that I'd crossed the line from a fat, overweight person to a *big* person. I'd moved from wearing "what looks good" to wearing whatever would fit, and that's not the type of woman I wanted to be. I thought, "I do not want to live like this, full of negative thinking and self-loathing, for another twenty-five years."

My biggest obstacle: All my life, bread has been my number-one enemy. When I was overweight, I would eat up to ten slices every night. Creamy yogurt would also get me into trouble. It was actually a relief when I realized those foods weren't in my food plan. Now, if I eat bread at all, I limit it to my breakfast, typically when I'm out at a restaurant (I won't keep it in my house). PJ also taught me it's not smart to ever reach for these binge foods if I am tired or alone.

At one point I hit a plateau and the scale wouldn't budge. PJ suggested I spend time visualizing myself in smaller clothes and seeing my tummy as toned and flat as possible. When I drove or pushed the grocery cart through the store, I'd picture myself fitting into a pair of fitted jeans and a cute T shirt rather than sweats. I also visualized that easy feeling of being able to quickly throw on an outfit and run out the door. All of these tools came together to help me reach my goal weight.

PJ's best advice: If there are fifty 50-year-old women standing in a line, I deserve to be in better shape and health than all of them. He also helped me eliminate dairy and use frozen vegetables to speed up meal preparation, and he showed me that just because a magazine or friend tells me a food is healthy, that doesn't mean it is. PJ emphasized the importance of a positive mental attitude and taught me to train hard every time, dedicating myself to just fifteen minutes of cardio but making it worthwhile.

ASH SACHDEV, age twenty-five

STARTING WEIGHT: 194 pounds
CURRENT WEIGHT: 176 pounds
POUNDS LOST: 18

Pounds away from goal weight: I'm more focused on body-fat loss. I started at 15 percent and want to get down to 8 percent.

Why I wanted to lose weight: I initially came to PJ to lose some weight before taking my first trip to Europe. My motivation was clear: I wanted to be able to take my shirt off at a beach and feel and look good. In the last ten years I can count on one hand how many times I have gone swimming or to the beach without a top on.

My biggest obstacle: My love of food. I looked forward to meals and tended to eat relatively healthy, but I didn't know when to say "enough." Through PJ I started to see this unhealthy food as a luxury you earn. I was also a diet-soda addict. I'd had two liters a week for the past seven years. PJ told me this was the first thing I had to stop because, although it is sugar-free, it is loaded with chemicals. The first week was tough, but I am proud to say it's been nine months without a soda—something I would have never thought possible. I immediately dropped five pounds and my sleep improved dramatically.

But my *biggest* obstacle is time to get everything done. I work an office job as an analyst from 8:30 a.m. to 7 p.m. most days. I used to find it very difficult to motivate myself to train after work; I was always tired and felt sluggish. Training with PJ has changed this; as a result of my new food plan and regular exercise, I have tons more energy and look forward to my workouts.

PJ's best advice: Don't worry about the past or about what anyone says.

During my first few weeks if I slipped up and ate badly, I would stress about it. PJ would ask me, "What's the point? It's in the past. Focus your energy instead on your next workout and your food plan for this week. You can't change the past, but you can change the future, so let's do this!"

SUZANNE KONSTANTINIDES, age forty-six

STARTING WEIGHT: 171 pounds
CURRENT WEIGHT: 138 pounds
POUNDS LOST: 33
POUNDS AWAY FROM GOAL WEIGHT: 10

Why I wanted to lose weight: To look, feel, and be healthy. I wanted to regain my confidence and know the feeling of having achieved something I never thought I could.

My biggest obstacle: Eating too much and not being able to stop. I lacked self-control and constantly craved carbohydrates as well as sweet and savory foods. Family gatherings would also make me feel anxious because everything is focused on food—and lots of it. PJ showed me how planning out my days, including what to eat and when, can help me stay on track.

PJ's best advice: Apart from the practical stuff, like eating clean, focusing on my workouts, planning meals, and believing in myself, the best advice he has given me deals with eating out at restaurants. He tells me to enjoy it, not feel guilty, and just get back on track the next day.

JOHN PARKES, MMBS (Australian MD), age sixty

STARTING WEIGHT: 257 pounds
CURRENT WEIGHT: 169 pounds
POUNDS LOST: 88
POUNDS AWAY FROM GOAL WEIGHT: 0—reached goal weight!

Why I wanted to lose weight: My blood pressure was up, requiring a number of medications. I was experiencing heart palpitations and became out of breath easily. I am a medical doctor, and I realized that I was encouraging patients to lose weight for their health, but I was not taking my own advice. I was talking the talk but not walking the walk. With my sixtieth birthday six months away, I knew that if I didn't take the necessary steps, I was setting myself up for a heart attack. I wanted to be around for my wife, my children, and my yet-to-come grandchildren—not die prematurely of some obesity-related disease.

My biggest obstacle: Before PJ my biggest obstacle to losing weight was giving my own weight loss and fitness priority in my busy life. PJ's encouragement helped me commit myself to his weight-loss and fitness way of life. He's wonderfully encouraging and empowering, he somehow manages to make training fun, and he makes me feel that I'm okay as a person—that I *can* do it and that I *will* get there. And I have!

PJ's best advice: There were two pieces of advice I really appreciated: "Don't worry about the weekly ups and downs of your weight; it's the long-term pattern that counts" and "Don't believe the myths about weight loss being more difficult if you're older or if you're nearing your goal; you will lose the weight regardless if you just keep with the KO-90 program."

ZOI GEORGIOU, age twenty-five

STARTING WEIGHT: 178 pounds
CURRENT WEIGHT: 123 pounds
POUNDS LOST: 55
POUNDS AWAY FROM GOAL WEIGHT: 0—reached goal weight!

Why I wanted to lose weight: I was just sick of hating my body; I couldn't even stand to look at myself in the mirror. Shopping with friends was the worst—after trying on five or six outfits, I'd have to lie and say that something fit me when really it didn't, because I was just embarrassed. My personal life was struggling because, when you feel horrible on the outside, you put up a shield and lie to yourself every day that it's okay to live an unhealthy lifestyle. You trick yourself into believing you are happy when actually you're miserable. I felt in my gut that I needed and wanted to turn my life around. That's what made me get up early every morning for training.

My biggest obstacle: Myself. My mentality was "It's impossible. There's no way I could ever have the body I want while also working a full-time job and enjoying a social life." I'd also had previous trainers label my goals as unattainable, so when PJ told me that I truly would drop the weight, I thought he was crazy!

PJ's best advice: Quit smoking. At first I didn't want to—I enjoyed it with my morning coffee—but I promised him I would, and I haven't had a cigarette for about twelve months now. It's probably the best thing I've ever done. I don't miss it, and in fact, I can't even stand being around it anymore!

SAM TRAD, age forty-four

STARTING WEIGHT: 224 pounds
CURRENT WEIGHT: 182 pounds
POUNDS LOST: 42
POUNDS AWAY FROM GOAL WEIGHT: 0—reached goal weight!

Why I wanted to lose weight: My main motivation for losing weight was to get fit and healthy. I wanted to be able to play football and soccer with my three young boys, but I lacked the energy and tired too easily. I also wanted to fit into regular clothes—especially fitted shirts. I was sick of wearing XL shirts that hung over my belly and looked like parachutes. Now I wear a medium or large, and my waistline went from 38 inches to 32.

My biggest obstacle was: I was too lazy and unmotivated. I'd typically start a sport and give up on it after two or three weeks. PJ would just keep motivating me and push me week after week—exactly what I needed.

PJ's best advice: Never give up and keep challenging yourself. He gave me a good, solid route to help me break old habits, and he trained me to eat the right food groups at the right times.

These clients are some of the most inspiring people I've ever met. True, they worked incredibly hard, and yes, they faced many obstacles and challenges along the way—ones that probably seem quite familiar to you. But they stuck with it and are now healthier and happier than they've ever been. I hope their stories—and my own—inspire you. Changing your life for the better only takes ninety days. Commit to the KO-90 program and put yourself on the road to the healthy life you've always wanted. The life you deserve!

ACKNOWLEDGMENTS

Firstly, I would like to thank my amazing fiancée, Lisa, who has been there for me every step of the way. Darling, thank you for your unwavering support, love, passion, and friendship. In you I have truly found my soulmate. I appreciate the hard work you have put in to help me with this book. I am grateful to you for everything you do for me on a daily basis. You are perfection personified!

Mum and dad, thank you for all that you have done over the years. Put simply, you are there for me each and every step of the way.

Many people have come together to create this book, and the following people have been directly responsible for the book being written and published.

To my agent, Steve Troha, at Folio Literary Management, this book has been made possible largely due to your belief in me. Thank you for your friendship, insight, and all your great advice along the way.

To my coauthor, Leslie Goldman, working together has been a very rewarding experience. From the outset we have gelled, and the result is a book of which I am very proud. Thank you for letting me ramble on about things without cutting me off. The process has been an absolute joy!

To my editor, Renee Sedliar, and the staff at Da Capo Press, thank you for believing in this book and placing your trust in me.

A big thank you to all my clients over the years. Each and every one of you has been a source of inspiration for me, and without you I wouldn't have the insight and knowledge to draw upon when writing this book. I never get tired of seeing a client transform into the person they never thought possible, the person they deserve to be.

A special mention goes to Davin Sgargetta and Aaron Carroll for following me from the very beginning and capturing my journey from fit to "Fat and Back" on film. You have worked tirelessly to ensure that the end result is exactly the way I envisaged it and more. Catching me in the gym late at night with a pizza that was about to be demolished after my first day back in "training" was extending me a lifeline. I wonder what may have happened if I wasn't caught red-handed!

To all my friends who have helped me with my journey from fit to "Fat and Back" and beyond, I appreciate you all very much, especially my close friend, Andrew Barlas. You are a true friend, and because of your handy camera work, my journey has also been captured in the form of daily photos. You placed your own life on hold to help me, and you encouraged me to believe that when it comes to eating, anything is possible! Putting on eighty-eight pounds in four months is quite simple; all you need is one person to choose the food and the other person to choose the quantity . . . now that's what I call teamwork!

To get my latest updates, you can follow me on:

Twitter: @pj_james
YouTube: www.youtube.com/pjfatandback
Website: www.paulPJjames.com

MY KO-90
PLAN JOURNAL

I WANT TO LOSE WEIGHT BECAUSE . . .

-
-
-
-
-

My before photo   My during photo   My after photo

WHAT I WANT/HOPE TO LOOK LIKE IN _____ MONTHS:

Measurements (initial and monthly)

Chest (measure at the nipple line)

_____

Waist (measure smallest part of your torso, usually a few inches above your navel)

_____

Hips (measure at the widest part, usually around the hip bones)

_____

Thighs (measure the widest part, usually just beneath your glutes)

_____

Calves

_____

Waist/hip ratio (initial and monthly)

_____

Heart rate/RHR (initial and monthly)

_____

Body-fat percentage (initial and monthly)

_____

One-minute time tests:

Push-ups (initial and monthly)

_____

Sit-ups (initial and monthly)

_____

Elliptical machine—distance covered in two minutes (initial and monthly);
(time taken to return to resting heart rate)

_____

The Plank Test—able to hold for _____ seconds (initial and monthly)

_____

TAKE IT OFF,

My KO-90 Workouts:

My KO-90 Shopping Lists:

TAKE IT OFF

NOTES

Introduction

1. American Society for Metabolic & Bariatric Surgery, "Obesity in America," ASMBS, http://www.asmbs.org/Newsite07/media/asmbs_fs_obesity.pdf.

2. FMI Research and Rodale/*Prevention*, "Shopping For Health 2010," Food Marketing Institute, 2010, http://www.fmi.org/forms/store/ProductFormPublic/search?action=1&Product_productNumber=2322; American Society for Metabolic & Bariatric Surgery, "Metabolic and Bariatric Surgery Overview," 2010, http://www.asmbs.org/Newsite07/media/ASMBS_Metabolic_Bariatric_Surgery_Overview_FINAL_09.pdf.

3. National Eating Disorders Association, "Fact Sheet on Eating Disorders," July 2010, http://www.nationaleatingdisorders.org/uploads/file/in-the-news/In%20the%20News%20Fact%20Sheet%20PDF.pdf.

4. Shaun Dreisbach, "Shocking Body-Image News: 97% of Women Will Be Cruel to Their Bodies Today," *Glamour*, February 2011, http://www.glamour.com/health-fitness/2011/02/shocking-body-image-news-97-percent-of-women-will-be-cruel-to-their-bodies-today.

Part 1

1. American Society for Metabolic & Bariatric Surgery, "Obesity in America," ASMBS, http://www.asmbs.org/Newsite07/media/asmbs_fs_obesity.pdf.

2. The National Institute of Mental Health, "Eating Disorders: Facts About Eating Disorders and the Search for Solutions," www.carf.org/WorkArea/DownloadAsset.aspx?id=22448.

3. "What Are the Guidelines for Percentage of Body Fat Loss?," American Council on Exercise, 2010, http://www.acefitness.org/blog/112/what-are-the-guidelines-for-percentage-of-body-fat/.

4. Joe Frascella, PhD, director of the Division of Clinical Neuroscience and Behavioral Research at National Institute on Drug Abuse in Bethesda, MD, interview, July 2009.

Part 2

1. Mark Bittman, "How to Make Oatmeal . . . Wrong," *New York Times*, February 22, 2011, http://opinionator.blogs.nytimes.com/2011/02/22/how-to-make-oatmeal-wrong/?partner=rss&emc=rss.

2. Karen Van Proeyen et al., "Training in the Fasted State Improves Glucose Tolerance during Fat-Rich Diet," *Journal of Physiology* 588, pt. 21 (November 2010): 4613–4614, http://jp.physoc.org/content/588/21/4289.abstract.

3. Obesity Education Initiative, "Clinical Guidelines on the Identification, Evaluation, and Treatment of Overweight and Obesity in Adults: The Evidence Report," 1998, http://www.nhlbi.nih.gov/guidelines/obesity/ob_gdlns.pdf.

4. Centers for Disease Control and Prevention, "Losing Weight," CDC, 2011, http://www.cdc.gov/healthyweight/losing_weight/index.html.

5. Sandra Gordon, "What Losing 10 Percent Can Do," 2011, http://www.weightwatchers.com/util/art/index_art.aspx?tabnum=1&art_id=41231&sc=3001.

6. Amy Berrington de Gonzalez et al., "Body-Mass Index and Mortality among 1.46 Million White Adults," *New England Journal of Medicine* 363, no. 23 (December 2010): 2211–2219, http://www.nejm.org/doi/full/10.1056/NEJMoa1000367.

7. "Obesity Increases Risk of Death in Severe Vehicle Crashes, Study Shows," *ScienceDaily*, December 21, 2010, http://www.sciencedaily.com/releases/2010/12/101221141106.htm.

8. Floriana S. Luppino et al., "Overweight, Obesity, and Depression: A Systematic Review and Meta-Analysis of Longitudinal Studies," *Archives of General Psychiatry* 67, no. 3 (2010): 220–229, http://archpsyc.ama-assn.org/cgi/content/abstract/67/3/220.

9. "Degree of Obesity Raises Risk of Stroke, Regardless of Gender, Race," *ScienceDaily*, January 21, 2010, http://www.sciencedaily.com/releases/2010/01/100121161236.htm.

10. "How Obesity Increases the Risk for Diabetes," *ScienceDaily*, June 21, 2009, http://www.sciencedaily.com/releases/2009/06/090621143236.htm.

11. National Institutes of Health, "Obesity in Men Linked to Infertility," *NIH News*, August 31, 2006, http://www.nih.gov/news/pr/aug2006/niehs-31.htm.

12. "A Missing Link from Obesity to Infertility Found," *EurekAlert!*, September 7, 2010, http://www.eurekalert.org/pub_releases/2010–09/cp-aml083110.php.

13. "Study Probes Obesity Link to Fibromyalgia," *ScienceDaily*, January 1, 2011, http://www.sciencedaily.com/releases/2010/12/101230113253.htm.

14. "Obesity Linked to Poor Colon Cancer Prognosis," *ScienceDaily*, March 11, 2010, http://www.sciencedaily.com/releases/2010/03/100309131752.htm.

15. H. Hampel, "Meta-Analysis: Obesity and the Risk for Gastroesophageal Reflux Disease and Its Complications," *Annals of Internal Medicine* 67, no. 3 (2005): 220–229, http://www.annals.org/content/143/3/199.

16. "Obesity—Mild or Severe—Raises Kidney Stone Risk," *ScienceDaily*, February 18, 2010, http://www.sciencedaily.com/releases/2010/02/100217182350.htm.

17. "Risk for Alcoholism Linked to Risk for Obesity," *ScienceDaily*, December 31, 2010, http://www.sciencedaily.com/releases/2010/12/101230172414.htm.

18. "Family, Friends, Social Ties Influence Weight Status in Young Adults," *ScienceDaily*, January 13, 2011, http://www.sciencedaily.com/releases/2011/01/110111133023.htm.

Part 3

1. A. Ariyo et al., "Depressive Symptoms and Risks of Coronary Heart Disease and Mortality in Elderly Americans," *Circulation* 102 (2000): 1773–1779, http://circ.ahajournals.org/cgi/content /full/102/15/1773.

2. E. Shackell and L. Standing, "Mind Over Matter: Mental Training Increases Physical Strength," *North American Journal of Psychology* 9, no. 1 (2007): 189–200, http://westallen.typepad .com/brains_on_purpose/files/mind_over_matter_shackell_07.pdf.

3. A. Geliebter and A. Aversa, "Emotional Eating in Overweight, Normal Weight, and Underweight Individuals," *Eating Behaviors* 3, no. 4 (January 2003): 341–347.

4. Judith J. Wurtman and Nina T. Frusztajer, *The Serotonin Power Diet: Eat Carbs—Nature's Own Appetite Suppressant—to Stop Emotional Overeating and Halt Antidepressant-Associated Weight Gain* (Emmaus, PA: Rodale Books, 2006).

5. Brian Wansink, "Is It a Brownie You Really Want? Or Just a Hug?," MSNBC, July 12, 2007, http://www.msnbc.msn.com/id/19174443/.

6. J. I. Hudson, E. Hiripi, H. G. Pope, and R. C. Kessler, "The Prevalence and Correlates of Eating Disorders in the National Comorbidity Survey Replication," *Biological Psychiatry* 61, no. 3 (February 2007): 348–358.

7. National Institute of Diabetes and Digestive and Kidney Diseases, "Binge Eating Disorder," Weight-control Information Network, 2008, http://www.win.niddk.nih.gov/publications/binge.htm.

8. Andrew Barr, "Graphic: How Big, Exactly, Is Starbucks' New 'Trenta' Size?" *National Post*, http://news.nationalpost.com/2011/01/17/graphic-how-big-exactly-is-starbucks-new-trenta-size/.

9. Obesity Education Initiative, "Clinical Guidelines on the Identification, Evaluation, and Treatment of Overweight and Obesity in Adults: The Evidence Report," 1998, http://www .nhlbi.nih.gov/guidelines/obesity/ob_gdlns.pdf.

10. P. M. Johnson and P. J. Kenny, "Corrigendum: Dopamine D2 Receptors In Addiction Like Reward Dysfunction and Compulsive Eating in Obese Rats," *Nature Neuroscience* 13, no. 5 (May 2010): 635–641.

11. Brian Wansink and Se-Bum. Park, "At the Movies: How External Cues and Perceived Taste Impact Consumption Volume," *Food Quality and Preference* 12, no. 1 (January 2001): 69–74.

12. B. Wansink and C. S. Wansink, "The Largest Last Supper: Depictions of Food Portions and Plate Size Increased Over the Millennium," *International Journal of Obesity* 34, no. 5 (May 2010): 943–944, http://www.nature.com/ijo/journal/vaop/ncurrent/full/ijo201037a.html.

13. N. A. Christakis and J. H. Fowler, "The Spread of Obesity in a Large Social Network over 32 Years," *New England Journal of Medicine* 357, no. 4 (July 26, 2007): 370–379.

14. S. Taheri, L. Lin, D. Austin, T. Young, and E. Mignot, "Short Sleep Duration Is Associated with Reduced Leptin, Elevated Ghrelin, and Increased Body Mass Index," *PLoS Medicine* 1, no. 3 (2004): e62.

Part 4

1. "NWCR Facts," The National Weight Control Registry, http://www.nwcr.ws/Research/default.htm.

2. Sharon P. Fowler, Ken Williams, Roy G. Resendez, Kelly J. Hunt, Helen P. Hazuda, and Michael P. Stern, "Fueling the Obesity Epidemic? Artificially Sweetened Beverage Use and Long-term Weight Gain," *Obesity* 16, no. 8 (2008): 1894–1900, http://www.nature.com/oby/journal/v16/n8/full/oby2008284a.html.

3. "Executive Summary," Center for Nutrition Policy and Promotion, http://www.cnpp.usda.gov/Publications/DietaryGuidelines/2010/PolicyDoc/ExecSumm.pdf.

4. Ian D. Stephen, Vinet Coetzee, and David I. Perrett, "Carotenoid and Melanin Pigment Coloration Affect Perceived Human Health," *Evolution and Human Behavior* (September 22, 2010), http://dx.doi.org/10.1016/j.evolhumbehav.2010.09.00.

5. "Dietary Reference Intakes: Water, Potassium, Sodium, Chloride, and Sulfate," Institute of Medicine (February 11, 2004), http://www.iom.edu/Reports/2004/Dietary-Reference-Intakes-Water-Potassium-Sodium-Chloride-and-Sulfate.aspx.

6. "Diet Sodas, Artificial Sweeteners Increase Waist Size, Blood Sugar Levels," *TopNews.in*, June 28, 2011, http://www.topnews.in/health/diet-sodas-artificial-sweeteners-increase-waist-size-blood-sugar-levels-212629.

7. "Waistlines in People, Glucose Levels in Mice Hint at Sweeteners' Effects: Related Studies Point to the Illusion of the Artificial," *ScienceDaily*, June 27, 2011, http://www.sciencedaily.com/releases/2011/06/110627183944.htm.

8. K. D. Vohs et al., "Making Choices Impairs Subsequent Self-Control: A Limited-Resource Account of Decision Making, Self-Regulation, and Active Initiative," *Journal of Personality and Social Psychology* 94, no. 5 (May 2008): 883–898, http://www.carlsonschool.umn.edu/assets/113144.pdf.

9. Division of Nutrition Research Coordination, "Do You Know Why You Eat?," National Institutes of Health, http://dnrc.nih.gov/pdf/nutritionmonth-brochure-08.pdf.

10. "Portion Distortion!," The National Heart, Lung, and Blood Institute, 2010, http://hp2010.nhlbihin.net/portion/index.htm.

11. "Yogurt Increases Fat Loss, UT Study Shows," The University of Tennessee, Knoxville, April 14, 2003, http://www.utk.edu/tntoday/2003/04/14/yogurt-increases-fat-loss-ut-study-shows/.

12. "Magnesium Supplements May Benefit People with Asthma," National Center for Complementary and Alternative Medicine, March 24, 2011, http://nccam.nih.gov/research/results/spotlight/021110.htm.

13. "Obesity Linked to Hormonal Changes, Lack of Sleep," Stanford University, December 8, 2004, http://news.stanford.edu/news/2004/december8/med-sleep-1208.html.

14. Julie Edgar, "Health Benefits of Green Tea," *Web MD*, May 26, 2010, http://www.webmd.com/food-recipes/features/health-benefits-of-green-tea.

15. S. Liu, W. C. Willett, J. E. Manson, F. B. Hu, B. Rosner, and G. Colditz, "Relation between Changes in Intakes of Dietary Fiber and Grain Products and Changes in Weight and Development of Obesity among Middle-Aged Women," *American Journal of Clinical Nutrition* 78, no. 5 (November 2003): 920–927, http://www.ncbi.nlm.nih.gov/sites/entrez?Db=pubmed&Cmd

=ShowDetailView&TermToSearch=14594777&ordinalpos=5&itool=EntrezSystem2.PEntrez
.Pubmed.Pubmed_ResultsPanel.Pubmed_RVDocSum.

16. J. W. Anderson, T. J. Hanna, X. Peng, and R. J. Kryscio, "Whole Grain Foods and Heart Disease Risk," *Journal of the American College of Nutrition* 19, no. 3 (June 2000): 291S–299S, http://www.jacn.org/cgi/reprint/19/suppl_3/291S.pdf.

17. P. Koh-Banerjee and E. B. Rimm, "Whole Grain Consumption and Weight Gain: A Review of the Epidemiological Evidence, Potential Mechanisms and Opportunities for Future Research," *Proceedings of the Nutrition Society* 62, no. 1 (February 2003): 25–29, http://www.ncbi.nlm.nih.gov/pubmed/12740053.

18. J. S. L. de Munter, F. B. Hu, D. Spiegelman, M. Franz, and R. M. van Dam, "Whole Grain, Bran, and Germ Intake and Risk of Type 2 Diabetes: A Prospective Cohort Study and Systematic Review," *PLoS Medicine* 4, no. 8 (2007): e261, http://www.plosmedicine.org/article/info:doi/10.1371/journal.pmed.0040261.

Part 5

1. E. G. Trapp, D. J. Chisholm, J. Freund, and S. H. Boutcher, "The Effects of High-Intensity Intermittent Exercise Training on Fat Loss and Fasting Insulin Levels of Young Women," *International Journal of Obesity* (2008): 1–8, http://www.med.unsw.edu.au/somsweb.nsf/resources/POM0801/$file/Jan08.pdf.

2. Timothy Heden, Curt Lox, Paul Rose, Steven Reid, and Erik P. Kirk, "One-Set Resistance Training Elevates Energy Expenditure for 72 h Similar to Three Sets," *European Journal of Applied Physiology* 111, no. 3 (2011): 477–484, http://www.springerlink.com/content/g85n7356577h7gq1/.

3. Ryan Bradley, "Resistance Isn't Always Futile: Strength Training in Diabetes," *Diabetes Action*, 2008, http://www.diabetesaction.org/site/PageServer?pagename=complementary_4_08.

INDEX

TAKE IT OFF,

TAKE IT OFF

TAKE IT OFF,

TAKE IT OFF,